THE
LOST LITERATURE
OF SOCIALISM

George Watson

We are still undegenerate in race; a race mingled of the best northern blood. We are not yet dissolute in temper, but still have the firmness to govern and the grace to obey.   John Ruskin, *Lectures on Art* (1870), inaugural

The great friendship after the great selection.   Leon Trotsky

*   In these sad times it is exceptionally comforting to see many Parisian workers talking to German soldiers as friends, in the street or at the corner café. Well done, comrades, and keep it up, even if it displeases some of the middle classes – as stupid as they are mischievous. The brotherhood of man will not remain forever a hope: it will become a living reality.*
                                        L'Humanité, 4 July 1940

The Lutterworth Press
Cambridge

for Robert Tombs

First Published in 1998 by:
The Lutterworth Press
P.O. Box 60
Cambridge
CB1 2NT
England

ISBN 0 7188 2983 2

British Library Cataloguing in Publication Data:
A catalogue record is available from the British Library.

Printed in England by
Redwood Books, Trowbridge

Contents

Acknowledgements

I am grateful to the University of São Paulo, Brazil for an invitation to deliver chapter 4 as a lecture, and to journals where earlier versions of four of these chapters, or rather parts of them, have appeared, notably *The Wilson Quarterly* (chapter 2), *History Today* (chapter 3), *Hudson Review* (chapter 5) and *Sewanee Review* (chapter 9); and to those who advised me how to improve them, as well as to a number of Polish and German libraries, especially the Jagellonian Library in Cracow, that helped me in my researches into National Socialism and its sources. The library of Lord Acton in the University Library of Cambridge, with his markings, has led me to such forgotten authors as Adolphe Franck and Alfred Sudre, on the last of whom the Ordre des Avocats à la Cour de Paris has generously provided fresh evidence.

But my most heartfelt thanks are due to the dedicatee, for inspiration as well as correction, and to the college that harbours us both.

Preface

The literature of socialism is lost in the sense that it is unread. At least most of it is, and this book is a report on what I have discovered by reading it.

It is the first account of socialist literature, I believe, since the defeat of Hitler, and certainly the first since the fall of the Wall in 1989. Being a study of a lost literature, it has little to say about justly famous books like *Fabian Essays* or Marx's *Capital*. Being essentially a literary study it is neither a comprehensive account of the socialist idea, like G.D.H. Cole's *A History of Socialist Thought* (1953-60) nor of Marxism, like Leszek Kolakowski's *Main Currents of Marxism* (1978) – still less a history of historical events and institutions such as the First, Second and Third Internationals or the October Revolution of 1917 – though, as so often with intellectual history, events keep breaking in, especially when genocide is in question. My object here is distinct. As a literary historian I seek to open doors to a new debate by studying revolution, class and race through largely forgotten texts in the hundred years or so that began in the 1840s, or the age that stretches from Marx to Hitler. This is a study in the unfamiliar. A lost literature is still a literature, after all, whether it survives in books, periodicals or manuscripts, and it is the business of the literary historian to read it.

Texts can surprise, especially when they are unread, and some of my conclusions may look startling. The first history of socialism, for example, a book unmentioned in any account of the subject, thought it a conservative idea. There is abundant evidence, some of which I produce in my early chapters, that socialism was not always supposed to be left-wing or favourable to the poor, whether by its adherents or its opponents. It was not always anti-racialist, what is more, and not always in favour of a welfare state. No one who reads the precursors of Marx – many of them Frenchmen of the 1840s – in addition to Marx himself, and no one who reads Ruskin and Morris, or Shaw, Wells, Tawney and Orwell, could imagine otherwise. In fact it is only as recently as the late 1930s, with the sudden emergence of the Popular Front in a dramatic, worldwide contest between fascism and communism, that socialism has been universally seen as wholly situated on the Left. As a great American humorist once said, it is better to know nothing than to know what ain't so.

This enquiry, then, is not an act of reverence; as befits the mood of the hour, it is revisionist. In 1992, after the fourth successive Labour defeat in a British general election, Roy Hattersley declared that the day of the sacred cow was done, and it is even becoming possible, at long last, to question the assumption that Left means virtue or that Right means competence. There has been too much conservative incompetence, and there have been too many socialist crimes, to make it easy by now to believe any such thing. All that admittedly makes for a perilous enterprise, since political convictions, in practice, are not plainly and simply a form of knowledge like botany or physics. They are more often a mode of self-definition, a claim to be a certain kind of being – caring if Left, competent if Right. In its heyday socialism was above everything a claim to virtue. You were not merely mistaken if you rejected it; you were at best a cynic and at worst a moral defective. A good deal will have to be unthought if, as I hope to show, the socialist tradition was once (among other things) conservative and genocidal, and unthinking can be harder than thinking and far more painful.

Any open-minded account of socialist literature, then, is likely to look like an act of irreverence. But there is one species of reverence to which, as a literary critic, I stand ever ready to plead guilty. I revere texts. Though not a socialist myself, I accept that the great socialist and anti-socialist thinkers of the past century and a half, voluminous and unstimulating as their works sometimes are, still deserve to be attentively read and scrupulously interpreted. That, surely, is why they wrote, and in this book I do them the honour of assuming that they said what they meant and meant what they said. When Marx and Engels publicly advocated genocide in 1849, for example, they did so because they wanted whole races to be killed. They were not ironising, sounding off or showing off. Or again, when the Labour leaders opposed William Beveridge's plans for a national health service, as he reports in *Power and Influence*, they did so because they were against it and because, as socialists, they believed they had good reasons to be against it. To humanise capitalism, after all, is to preserve it, and subsequent events do not suggest that their fears were misplaced. Socialist governments in more recent years that have set out to dismantle state welfare should not be thought of as behaving in untraditional ways.

In a word, I study texts for what they have to say. If some find that a sadly literal view, I can only reply that literature is above all interesting for what it says, and that if it were supposed to tell us nothing but what we already believed, or wanted to believe, it would have lost all its power to change mankind.

St John's College
Cambridge

1
A Literature Lost

The socialist idea spans a century and a half, in round terms, starting in the 1840s.

Its literary sources, however, reach back into the last years of the eighteenth-century Enlightenment, when revolution (it is strange to tell) first became a radical word and when theories of social difference began their continuous life. Without revolution and class, the story cannot be told. So this book is about the gestation of socialism as well as its life – a study of origins and sources as well as of triumph and decay.

The literature of a political idea that lasted for less than two centuries looks manageable as a theme, for an historian or a political scientist. I am neither, and it may be asked why a literary critic, of all people, would choose to deal with it or expect to be heeded if he did. The answer lies in seeking out texts and reading them. Some authors are by now wholly obscure and forgotten. To read them, or the less famous works of famous men, is to attend to what they say rather than to what they are traditionally supposed to have said or to what their modern disciples wish they had said. 'The struggle of man against power', as Milan Kundera proclaims, 'is the struggle of memory against forgetting'.

That is the task. The critical mind tests traditional assumptions to destruction, if it is dutiful and alert, and instinctively distrusts anything that looks or smells like a received idea. It is a task that can make enemies as well as friends. By an odd reversal, the Left in recent years has grown more fearful of innovation than those who call themselves conservatives, as if its defensive postures in matters of state – no cuts, no pit closures – had entered into its habits of thinking about the socialist past. Time, which looked to be on its side a century ago and more when Bernard Shaw edited *Fabian Essays*, is no longer that, as it knows, and it can easily take offence at any hint of blasphemy against its canon of saints or alarm at the thought of what the socialist pioneers, in the last century and this, may have said or done. By the mid-twentieth century the intellectual Left had turned nervously reverential and conformist, muttering to itself sacred names like Chartism and the Tolpuddle Martyrs, Walter Benjamin and Bertolt Brecht – and above all Lenin, who, as a recent historian of the Russian Revolution has remarked, became after his death in 1924 the object of a hagiography strongly messianic in flavour: 'self-denying devotion to the cause, modesty, self-discipline, generosity', his life being modelled on the life of Christ.[1] Christology was seldom far distant from the socialist idea and, always state-centred, it was ideally suited to become an established religion. In the classic shift from subversion to orthodoxy few doctrines can have had so little distance to travel.

By the 1960s – if not earlier – it had become impious in the western world to probe into what the fathers of the faith were once supposed to have believed. That reverent mood was well caught by J.G. Merquior in *Western Marxism*, where as an ex-Marxist he delicately and remorselessly exposed the philosophical pretensions of recent academic and semi-academic theorising about social history and the sociology of thought. The book was a brave one, since the philosophy of socialism had by then become something like a no-go area for the faithful, rather like the inner sanctum of a temple cult; and anyone who wants to understand piety would do better to read back-numbers of the *New Left Review* than the *Church Times*. There were things which, in the heyday of the Left, one was simply not supposed to mention, like the idea of conservative revolution, the early resistance of socialist leaders to the welfare state, or the openly Tory allegiance of early socialists, some of whom were proud to declare Toryism their chief reason for being what they were. Public ownership, after all, was always a demand to make the biggest capitalist of all bigger still. Who, for that matter, cared to remember the long socialist tradition of racial discrimination and genocide? In the writing of history what men choose to forget is as significant as what they strive to remember.

Impiety, then, seems inevitable here, and it is a prospect calculated to stimulate and embolden. This is autopsy-time. It is part of the proper business of the critic, after all, to be impious, and if I invade the territory of political thought here, and not for the first time, it is in the sober conviction that the writings even of the famous are little studied and seldom pondered. The very names of some notable theorists have now wholly faded from view. There are still social historians who take it for granted, for example, that comprehensive theories of social difference began with Marx, though Marx himself did not think so. For this reason I have devoted a chapter to John Millar's *Origin of the Distinction of Ranks* of 1771, unsocialist though it is, since it is the first theoretical book on the subject in all Europe and a work now utterly passed out of mind; another to a neglected aspect of Tocqueville's view, as an early liberal, of the dangers to liberty inherent in social equality; another to the Tory tradition of socialism in the last century and this, since there were always socialists who hated progress and demanded a return to ancient values. It is a myth born of incuriosity to suppose they invariably thought of themselves as

---

1. Richard Pipes, *The Russian Revolution 1899-1919*, pp. 341, 345.

left-wing; from first to last there were socialists who believed in a privileged class and said so, and the fat privileges of the Soviet *nomenklatura* were not an unpredicted or unintended consequence of Lenin's seizure of power in 1917. It was admirably candid of Todor Zhivkov, the former Communist dictator of Bulgaria, to admit at his trial in Sofia in February 1991 that his large gifts to friends and relatives were normal socialist practice. 'This was the situation in all socialist countries', he said. And so it was.

The neglect of texts in political theory is remarkable, as the fate of John Millar's book illustrates. Or of Alfred Sudre's *Histoire du Communisme* – the first history of the subject in any language, and a work now so little known that I have yet to find anyone in France, or anywhere, who has so much as heard of it, though it won a prize from the French Academy when it first appeared, went through several editions and translations, and bristles with acute observations and pertinent predictions. Composed by a young Parisian lawyer who had just taken part in the revolution of 1848, it does not even mention Marx or Engels; so the tradition of communism, as Marx and Engels knew, is older than the *Communist Manifesto* of 1848 – though perhaps not as old, as Sudre implies in his thoughtful book, as Plato or Sir Thomas More. The socialist tradition of racial extermination, again, though it was touched on fleetingly in F.A. Hayek's *The Road to Serfdom* in 1944, is now so seldom mentioned that even experts can look blankly incredulous to be told of it, and I have known some to look blank even after works by Marx and Engels, Shaw and Wells, are quoted to them. The very titles are largely unfamiliar. Who, after all, has read H.G. Wells's *Anticipations* of 1902, which in its last pages calls on a socialist utopia to destroy the 'grey confusion' of democracy through a world state governed by a self-appointed white élite that would purify mankind by exterminating the dark races? Wells's aim was efficiency, and part of a long tradition of socialist genocide and white-supremacy doctrines spanning two centuries; as Michael Coren implied in *The Invisible Man* in 1993, he was part of a long tradition. 'The world is a world, not a charitable institution', Wells wrote grimly in his concluding pages, demanding genocide. When Hitler called his movement National Socialism, the title was widely condemned by German socialist parties as a deceitful manoeuvre secretly inspired by high finance, but its racial policies, for good reason, were not seen as unsocialist. The real objection to communist ideas, Hitler once told a confidant, is that 'basically they are not socialist', since they create mere herds without individual life.

This book seeks to lift layers of whitewash, and it is prompted by the conviction that the texts of socialism, for and against, are often simply unread and even unheard of, and are surprising enough, in consequence, to repay attention. It is about a lost literature – at times, one feels, an

embarrassing literature, a literature deliberately lost. 'Some people', said
Mao Tse-Tung in a speech of March 1957 – it is penultimate among his
Thoughts – 'have read a few Marxist books and think themselves quite
learned, but what they have read has not penetrated, has not stuck in their
minds'. That sounds like a job for a literary critic to do: it involves
rediscovering a body of texts, reading them and paying attention to them.
In 1992 a Conservative prime minister in the flush of victory called
socialism a museum-piece. If so, it is like a medal that has lain in a locked
case for a century and more, and no one has troubled to turn it over. It is
time somebody did.

The present case, however, it must be confessed at the outset, represents
a highly exceptional and puzzling instance of how a literature can get lost
and stay lost. Socialism was always a scriptural doctrine, after all, in the
sense of being avowedly based on famous texts: texts almost always
available, and for long periods compulsory reading for hundreds of millions
in eastern Europe and Asia. There are three historical phases here, and my
emphasis will fall largely on the first, the age of conception from the 1840s
to 1917. It was followed by an age of fulfilment culminating in theCommunist
seizure of power in China in 1949, and an age of decline that ended with
the fall of the Wall in 1989. Oddly enough, the age of fulfilment (1917-
49) was also one of neglect, in the sense that it engendered a mood in
which socialism was widely venerated and little studied. Perhaps it was
studied so little because it was venerated so much. Anyone who has spent
a lifetime working in universities will know how widely, in that age and
for years after, it was a word held to sanctify argument and silence debate.
There were always anti-socialists. But they were supposed to be sceptics
and cynics, and the possibility of a radical, idealistic anti-socialism has
never quite taken root in the western mind. Even among its enemiessocialism
is still widely believed to have been a generous and benevolent notionfatally
flawed by a set of technical difficulties which its disciples, by someoversight,
highmindedly failed to predict. This book is designed to destroy that myth.

To a literary historian the world of political history must always look
surprising. Historians of political thought are no doubt aware that great
thinkers of past ages wrote books; but they often seem strikingly incurious
about what is in them. That paradox will emerge in the pages that follow.
The first history of socialism, for example, which thought it a conservative
idea, was promptly dismissed by Proudhon in about 1850 as a mass of
platitudes; but nobody a century later would have thought it platitudinous
to call socialism conservative, which shows what a short life platitudes
can have. In a letter of July 1864 Gustave Flaubert, who was reading
socialist authors like Charles Fourier at the time with a view to writing his
novel *L'Éducation Sentimentale*, complained that he felt weighed down

by the tedium of the task. Socialist writers were authoritarian and boorish, he complained (*despotes et rustres*), their reactionary minds stuck in the Middle Ages, and obsessed with class or caste consciousness (*l'esprit de caste*), with hardly anything in common, what is more, except a hatred of liberty and of the French Revolution. It was like doing the dreariest school-work: 'Le socialisme moderne pue le pion'. By mid-century it was not unusual to see socialism as backward-looking and snobbish; and the author of *Madame Bovary*, a connoisseur equally of tedium and of class-consciousness, does not sound much surprised by what he found.

His impatience was natural. A critic of any age – it must be conceded at once – and of any persuasion, would hesitate to make high artistic claims for much of the literature of socialism. What can be said in its favour can be quickly said. With *The Communist Manifesto* of 1848 Marx wrote a good pamphlet, and among English authors Bernard Shaw and H.G. Wells are plainly readable; so are some novelists and poets, French and English, of the 1930s. But the dust grows thick on most of these works, and perhaps the nearest approach to a great socialist novel in any language remains *The Man of Property*, the first volume of the *Forsyte Saga*, where John Galsworthy deftly illustrated the destructive ethos of an owning class through the tragedy of an unhappy marriage, where a sense of material possession destroys love.

As their most ardent admirers would probably agree, what is more, the classics of socialism do not usually demand great subtlety of interpretation. In an enthusiastic article called "The literary achievement of Marx" which she wrote for *Modern Quarterly* (1947), Pamela Hansford Johnson praised his style as richly characterised by Gothic imagery and a 'cleansing anger', but seldom if ever by obscurity. Even Marx's irony, as she saw – while confessing that she had read him only in translation – is an irony instantly decipherable: 'always uncomfortable, never ambiguous'. That is an apt and significant point, the more so since it is not a judgement one would make of the political writings of the eighteenth-century Enlightenment or of its liberal heirs in the nineteenth century and since; nor of such conservative thinkers as Benjamin Disraeli or Michael Oakeshott. Socialist literature may not always be a joy to read, but it commonly leaves the interpreter little to do. But then it believed, in its heyday, that the world around it – the capitalist world – was just about to end, and that is a conviction unlikely to encourage the graces of art.

Even sex, it is surprising to report, seldom succeeds in animating the writings of the socialists. Charles Fourier, of whose style Flaubert complained, died as early as 1837, and was best known for inventing the phalanstery – a rural community ideally of 1,620 people – where life, labour and its rewards were to be governed by elaborate rules. At his death he left a manuscript called *Le Nouveau Monde Amoureux*, composed in 1817-18, a utopia in the pre-Marxian vein composed at a time when other radicals, like Shelley, were interesting themselves in free love. Fourier sought to harmonise the passions and instincts of mankind by releasing them from repression, which he saw as the source of such perversities as sadism and homosexuality, and by linking sexual urges to the movements of the heavenly bodies. Unknown to Flaubert, the book lay unpublished in five notebooks until 1967, a time that might be thought propitious to a theory of sexual freedom and social revolution, but in the event it went largely unnoticed. Even free love, it seems, does not survive long stretches of socialist prose.

The conservatism of the socialist idea was familiar to at least some Victorians as an argumentative point. That familiarity, however, did not last. Utopias are evidently characterised by the brevity of their shelf-life, and there seem to be truths that each generation has to discover for itself. When George Orwell and Arthur Koestler revived the point in the 1940s they made no reference whatever to the Victorian debate, and it seems clear that they believed they had discovered it for themselves. A generation later, however, in the 1960s, the essential conservatism of socialism had been forgotten all over again, and it was almost universally believed that it had never been thought of as anything but left-wing. It is hard to judge how much here is indolence, how much suppression. Dull as the materials often are, there must also have been a refusal to look – an ideological refusal all the easier to maintain because there were so few literary master-pieces demanding to be read. But if the Tory and genocidal traditions of socialism have been suppressed rather than forgotten, then this must count as one of the most successful acts of suppression in intellectual history; and a considered challenge to such incuriosity, whatever its motives, was bound in the end to be made.

The paradox of a literature at once venerated and forgotten must remain forever striking, and the paradox was there as early as the nineteenth century. When William Morris joined the Social Democratic Federation in 1883, as he explained in "How I became a socialist", he had 'never so much as opened Adam Smith, or heard of Ricardo or Karl Marx', though he later managed to read and enjoy the historical parts of Marx's *Capital*.[1] But then socialism, for Morris, bluntly meant 'equality of condition', which he would not have found in Marx. H.G. Wells, meanwhile, who once boasted an irreverent desire to see Marx shaved, claimed in *Russia in the Shadows* (1920) that he was already a complete Marxist by the age of fourteen, which was in 1880, and 'long before I had heard the name of

---

1. *Justice* (16 June 1894), reprinted in William Morris, *Political Writings,* p. 242

Marx'; so that Marx, who died in 1883, seems even in his lifetime to have joined that distinguished band of authors – Machiavelli and Freud are perhaps other instances – whose works are felt to be understood without acquaintance. Shortly after the infant Wells, if he is to be believed, had thought of Marxism without any help from Marx, the young Bernard Shaw went to a London meeting of H.M. Hyndman's Social Democratic Federation. That, as he tells in "How I became a public speaker" in *Sixteen Self Sketches* (1949), was in 1884, while he was still in his twenties. He was 'contemptuously dismissed as a novice who had not read the great first volume of Marx's *Capital*'. So he promptly read it in a French translation in the British Museum and joined the Fabian Society. 'Immediately contempt changed to awe; for Hyndman's disciples had not read the book themselves.' That set a pattern destined to continue, and it seems clear that in the realm of political theory it is not reading that most commonly converts. Raymond Williams would freely admit that he belonged to a generation that read very little Marx, implying perhaps that he thought other generations read a lot of him, and in a radio interview Eric Hobsbawm has recently told how, as a schoolboy in pre-Hitler Berlin, he became a Marxist without reading a word of him, and how he only began reading him at all because his schoolmaster told him he did not know what he was talking about. In *Starting Out in the Thirties* (1966), similarly, Alfred Kazin has revealed of his teenage self that socialism in those early years was 'a way of life', since 'everyone else I knew in New York was a socialist, more or less'. No other view was heard. Socialism was not a gesture of revolt but an unthinking act of conformity, and reading had nothing to do with it. It is always rash to assume that intellectuals admire only authors they know.

In the 1950s and 1960s, when socialism ruled a third of the human race, vast portraits of Marx, Engels, Lenin, Stalin and Mao, all of them voluminous authors, adorned public festivities in the Soviet empire and China – they were jocularly known as the Decline of the Beard – and the *Thoughts* of Mao Tse-Tung was a best-seller that easily outran, for a time, the Bible and *The Pilgrim's Progress*. But who, even among the most earnest disciples or dedicated opponents, ever read more than the tiniest percentage of what they wrote? Then confirmation came, and it was swift and terrible. In 1992 literary Paris was startled and shocked by the posthumous autobiography of Louis Althusser, *L'Avenir Dure Longtemps*, where one of the most internationally celebrated of academic Marxists revealed that he had read hardly any of the writings he had been expounding as a philosopher in Paris for decades: not a word of Aristotle or Kant, for example, though he had lectured on them, and among Marx's own writings only the early works. The author of *Lire le Capital* (1968) had not read *Das Kapital*.

The case, on reflection, looks unique. The great scriptural religions, after all, like Christianity and Islam, do not behave in that carefree way: they study their scriptures and squabble about interpreting them, and those squabbles are creditable to the extent that they demonstrate that reading is done and attention paid. Literary cults like Homer and Shakespeare, too, are based on reading and rereading, generation by generation and in the original texts, so that religion and literature both set commendable examples of attention-giving. It may be worth asking, then, why political theorists seldom behave in that way.

One provisional answer may be that theories of politics, even more quickly than religious dogmas, can ossify into positions held and proclaimed by groups, parties and interests; and like the easy assumption that socialism was always left-wing, they can rapidly entrench into slogans that come to represent institutions, mass parties and ruling élites. Giving them up can mean giving up the certitudes of a lifetime and everything that follows from those certitudes, which can include acquaintances and friends. It is a phenomenon called the Tyranny of the Terms. Few modern theorists have shared H.G. Wells's impious and outspoken ambition to see Marx shaved. It is an alarming thought. What is more, in France and Italy the terms Left and Right – in the English-speaking world largely the property of intellectuals – are common change in ordinary conversation and newspaper headlines to signify socialist and anti-socialist, so that some highly disabling assumptions are by now buried deep in the day-to-day usage of the ignorant as well as the learned. These assumptions are not to be questioned lightly, and it can look cranky, or worse, to question them at all.

A despair that one may never be read at all can afflict the very act of writing. Who, if anyone, is listening? In 1901, for example, Max Hirsch (1852-1909), a Prussian disciple of Henry George who in 1890 had settled in Australia, completed an extensive book called *Democracy versus Socialism* which he believed to be the first comprehensive refutation of socialism ever published. A radical himself, he saw socialism as the road to slavery, promising only 'an all-pervading despotism' by a new managerial class. That was nearly half a century before George Orwell's *Animal Farm*. But Hirsch's preface, characteristically, holds out no realistic hope that his warning against tyranny will be heeded. That is because socialists cannot listen. Confident in their conviction that social reform can only mean socialism, they are 'deaf'. It is a book which, appearing in the first year of the twentieth century, sums up an age to come. Anti-socialists do not quote it; Orwell and Koestler, a generation on, do not appear to have known of its existence. It is a warning unheard.

By the later years of the twentieth century it was not only, or even mainly, the Left that would not listen. Deafness had become a nearly universal complaint. Conservatives too could feel they had a lot to lose from a revival of interest in socialism as a conservative regression to ancient values. A dud theory, what is more, made an ideal opposition. 'Whatever have the Conservatives done', a wit remarked after the 1983 British election, when Labour under Michael Foot lost disastrously on a socialist programme, 'to deserve the Labour party?' The Left-and-Right game, by then, looked like a game too good to spoil, and anyone who questioned it had about as much chance of a hearing as an outsider to Oxford and Cambridge who called for a third team in the Boat Race. The conviction, above all, that socialism was always about class and never about race – that it cannot, for that simple reason, have advocated genocide – has been a near-universal illusion for decades. Conservatives have been as ready to accept it as socialists, and if the exclusive association of socialism with the Left had depended on socialists alone it would not have survived as sturdily as it did and does.

That world of assumption, it is now clear, was a superstitious world, in the sense of being indifferent to evidence and content to remain so. Samuel Johnson once remarked that there are superstitions not connected with religion, and anyone who has studied the recent history of political ideas is bound to be vividly aware of it. The significant contrast here is between Left and Radical. Left can easily be a cosy and self-consoling state of mind – a middle-class way of looking and feeling unguilty about a privileged upbringing – whereas the radical mind, by contrast, stands ready to doubt and question the assumptions common to debate. It would not occur to the Left, for example, to ask whether socialism is or always was left-wing: to the radical it is among the first of questions to be asked. Some of these chapters, accordingly, concern a contrast of individuals who illustrate the spiritual consolations of the Left, on the one hand, and the disturbing power of minds as radical as Tocqueville's and Orwell's on the other. Who now cares to recall that the British Conservative Party was once the chief anti-competitive party in Britain, dedicated, above everything, to protectionism, high spending, taxation and centralised power? Its hallmark, as John Stuart Mill remarked in a letter of October 1831, was 'a reverence for government in the abstract' and a deep conviction that it is 'good for a man to be ruled'. No wonder socialists often found themselves closer to conservatives than to liberals. Some, like John Ruskin, even called themselves Tories or King's Men, and it was only as recently as the 1970s that British Tories began belatedly to discover the virtues of the free market.

To dig is to find treasure, and some of the notions of the early socialists may be found worth reviving on their merits. No one, after all, has ever demonstrated any conservative social effects to a competitive free market, or any necessary or probable connection between centralised economic planning and the abolition of poverty; and there was always plenty in socialist doctrine to attract the aristocratic temperament and established interests, as the struggle of conservative communists against Boris Yeltsin in the Russian Federation has recently illustrated. Socialism could even mean a new style of royalism, for some, provoked by an industrial revolution and a fearful memory of the Terror.

Perhaps the first instance of royal socialism, and certainly the most improbable, was Queen Victoria's father, the Duke of Kent, one of George III's sons, though he belongs to the prehistory of the doctrine, since he died in January 1820 before the word was invented. In his autobiographical *Life* (1857) Robert Owen, the socialist pioneer, proudly tells how the Duke had openly admired his principles and called for 'a much more just equality' than any that yet existed – one that would 'give much more security and happiness to all than the present system can give to any'. The formula hints at a benevolence spurred by fear – a rational fear entirely natural to the great European aristocracies as the Napoleonic wars drew to an end. Socialism in that age could look like a preservative and prudent act. At all events, the Duke of Kent was as much devoted to Robert Owen himself, if Owen's own account is to be believed, as to his ideas, and with an impressive assiduity chaired a committee dedicated to promoting his *New View of Society* (1813-16). That is a striking fact, even granting a circumstance Owen does not trouble to mention: that the Duke owed him money he could not repay. But the Duke of Kent has no great reputation as a hypocrite, and if he had lived to be king, as he hoped and expected, he might now be remembered as the first socialist monarch in Europe. Instead he took his family, including his infant daughter Victoria, to winter on the Devon coast, and died of an inflammation of the lungs a few days before the king his father.

The claim to be called the first socialist monarch, accordingly, belongs, a little uncertainly, to the Emperor Napoleon III of France, nephew of the first Napoleon and son of a king of Holland. The Napoleonic idea, as he understood it, was a heady cocktail of military glory abroad and a centralised administration at home under a command economy. His early life as an agitator under the July monarchy (1830-48), which imprisoned him, had led him into authorship, and his doctrinal position is fully known. A democracy needs central administration even more than an aristocratic government, he announced in his mid-thirties, in *Les Idées Napoléoniennes* (1839) – Lord Acton, in his copy of the book now in Cambridge, has pencilled a large question-mark here in the margin – and the state, rightly considered, is not a necessary ulcer, as an economist had recently put it, or a mere drain on wealth, but rather the beneficent impulse of every social organism that there is. Populist centralism perhaps takes its rise here. Composed in exile in England and published in Brussels and London as well as in Paris a dozen years before Louis Napoleon came to power in France, the book abounds in extravagant praise of his uncle Napoleon I, who not only achieved conquests abroad but rationalised old enterprises at home and founded new ones. True, it is not a socialist book, and it would be surprising if its author, as early as 1839, had heard of the word. He appears to know nothing of the doctrine of class struggle, in any case, and the work reeks of patriotism in the flamboyant style of the First Empire. But in its insistence on a centralised economy in the service of the poor it is a book calculated to create an atmosphere in which, in the 1840s and after, the nascent idea of socialism might begin to thrive; and in 1844, in prison, he wrote and published a pamphlet called *Extinction du Paupérisme* where he advocated distributing uncultivated land to the poor at public expense. Since his death Napoleon III has never been thought a hero of the Left, in spite of tolerating trade unions in 1864 six years before his defeat and deposition. But his enemies sometimes called him a socialist, and he reportedly called himself one. 'How can you expect my government to get on?' he once exclaimed half-seriously to a friend:

The Empress is a legitimist; Morny is an Orleanist; Prince Napoleon is a republican; I am a socialist . . . ; only Persigny is an Imperialist – and he is mad![1]

One refreshing mood in which to approach the past of socialism might be to accept that an emperor could think of himself as a socialist and be thought of as one; and certainly Napoleon III was not the last socialist ruler to dignify himself with the trappings of royalty. In February 1864, just before he was killed in a duel, Ferdinand Lassalle wrote to a friend that he had 'come to the conviction that nothing could have a greater future, or a more beneficent role, than monarchy, if it could only make up its mind to be a social monarchy'. That sounds much like the vision of Queen Victoria's father and of Napoleon III.

The royalism of the socialist idea was sometimes evident, what is more, to its sturdiest opponents. T.S. Eliot was one. Fresh from his year in Paris in 1910-11, where he had known French legitimists, and lecturing in London as a young American in 1916, he remarked approvingly, as one who had always been a conservative, that 'contemporary socialism has much in common with royalism';[2] and his recent involvement in Paris in the world of the Action Française, which was violently seeking to restore

---

1. Alix de Janzé, *Berryer,* p. 64
2. Ronald Schuchard, "T.S. Eliot as an extension lecturer 1916-1919", in *Review of English Studies 25,* (1974) p.166

the French monarchy, does not seem to have made him think the notion a
paradoxical one. Like conservatism, socialism sought to justify the state
anew and to reinstate in democratic and industrial societies the vital and
vanishing principle of subordination through regulation and planning. As
Mill said, there are those who think it is good for a man to be ruled.

That mood is perhaps hard to recover, and by now it is easy to look origi-
nal and even provocative by repeating truths that many Victorians would
have thought too familiar to be worth emphasising. Repetition can be pain-
ful. Few discoveries, as Lord Acton once remarked, are more irritating
than those that expose the pedigree of an idea. To rediscover the essential
royalism of the socialist idea means reading texts more than a century old
– often forgotten texts – and paying attention, and here the modern interpret-
er may find himself in a dilemma. If he notes only a few, like Napoleon III,
Lassalle and T.S. Eliot, he may be accused of contenting himself with the
occasional whimsies of famous men unscrupulously torn out of context; if
he notes many, of the pedant's besetting vice of overkill. But a least the
charge of overkill suggests that a point has been taken, however reluct-
antly, and faced with a familiar scholarly dilemma I have preferred here to
be accused of that.
    On a long view, then, this book should not be seen as original, or meant
to be. It is about what was widely thought and said over the course of a
century and more. An act of revival, not of innovation, it commemorates
great and sometimes forgotten names, socialist and other, who have argued
the case for and against revolution, class, equality and progress, and it
appears at a moment – the first in Europe since the Enlightenment – when
there are no fashionable ideologies or political gods, when the skies are
suddenly empty of saints and messiahs. My motive is to revive argument
in a sceptical and thoughtful age and to enrich and enliven a tradition
which, with the sudden Soviet collapse of 1989 and the slow decay of the
New Left, has fallen into disrepute and perhaps terminal decline. The
socialist idea now needs to be rescued from the failing grasp of moralists
who have left it with an unenviable reputation for woolly idealism and
endless priggery. In its day it was more complex and interesting than that.
It was not always dedicated to ideals of progress or hostile, in principle, to
racialism, monarchy, or aristocratic rule; it was not always a playground
for prigs. It may not have worked, as a doctrine, but it is worth more than
a wave of goodbye. One of the more imposing phenomena of modern
intellectual history, it once excited advocacy and defiance in some lively
intelligences and passionate hearts. It is richer and more various than we
know.

2
Millar or Marx?

There was once a professor of law called John Millar. Born in Scotland in 1735, he went to Adam Smith's lectures on moral philosophy and then, finding his own religious convictions too weak for a clerical career even in an age as sceptical as the Enlightenment, took to the law. In 1761 he became a professor at Glasgow, where he is said to have been among the first to lecture in English rather than Latin, acquiring an enviable reputation as an orator in his university and beyond. In the 1770s, as a militant Whig, he openly supported the American Revolution, and a dozen years later the French, and he opposed the slave trade.

He also wrote a treatise on social differences. His first book, it appeared in 1771, and in later editions came to be known as *The Origin of the Distinction of Ranks*: a work by a professor still in his thirties that plainly owed something to Montesquieu and to David Hume who (though a Tory) was a close friend. It is not now famous, and it has not been reprinted since 1806. In 1923, in a memorial volume for Max Weber called *Hauptprobleme der Soziologie*, Werner Sombart called it astonishing, altogether one of the best and most complete of sociologies, and wondered why it had dropped from view. In fact it was not widely celebrated even in its own century, and Boswell and Johnson do not mention it. Yet it was probably the first book in Europe to be devoted to the theory of social difference, and almost the only one in the western world before the present century.

Millar's invisibility since his death in 1801 is faintly surprising. He belonged, as a Scot, to a modest nation but not, as a lawyer, to a modest profession. His book went into several editions in his lifetime, with improvements, and was translated into German a year after it first appeared, and later into French; and there was even a Basel edition in the original English in 1793. But nineteenth-century theorists like Karl Marx seldom if ever mention it, though David Ricardo owned a copy and John Stuart Mill and his father James are known to have admired it, and it is now essentially unread and forgotten. In *The Enlightenment* (1969) Peter Gay allows several pages to Millar's views on slavery, but he seems to have no reputation as a sociologist; and it is now widely assumed, even by anti-Marxists, that modern theorising about social difference, and even social history itself, began in the 1840s with Marx and Engels. 'We are all Marxists now', a professor of classics remarked recently at an international conference, meaning no more than that ancient historians nowadays are interested above all in social history. Soon after the fall of communism, in 1991, an article called "Premature obsequies?" in *History Today*, by Christopher Hill, argued that Marxism is immortal even if the Soviet system was not, being conceptually indispensable to historians, and the argument has become a convenient bolt-hole for old comrades and can be unthinkingly accepted, at times, even by the non-political. A myth is being born, and it has two aspects: that social difference is always and necessarily the same as social class, and that theories of class began with Marx. These are enormous assumptions. I want to argue here that one can be intelligently interested in the theory of social difference without being interested in class at all – by rejecting, indeed, theories of class – and that the theoretical issue was at least a century old in modern Europe when Marx began to write about it in the 1840s: that Marx was a latecomer, in fact, to the debate, that he knew that he was, and that it was not improved by his intervention.

In 1748, exactly a century before the *Communist Manifesto* of Marx and Engels, Montesquieu's *Esprit des lois* appeared, a comparative study of human society that drew excited attention to how social institutions differ according to period, custom and climate. Montesquieu sought to reform the French monarchical system. He was neither a revolutionary nor a moral relativist, though this did not save his book from the papal index; in fact his first chapter insisted that the laws of life are given. God, he argues,

acts according to the laws of the universe because He knows them; knows them because He made them, made them because they are about wisdom and power,

every human and physical variation representing an ultimate uniformity, he insists, every change an ultimate consistency in human nature. Anthropology, in its infancy, did not entail the view that morality was a human invention or that it only exists relative to time and place. Moral laws are given, in that view, like physical laws; individuals and communities can get them right or wrong. Millar believed that too. Though his book is a study of the diversity of human customs, invoking Arabs, American Indians and even Congolese, its preface restates the foundation-doctrine of humanism that human nature is 'every where the same'; so that he is a disciple of Montesquieu's doctrine that diversities of sex, wealth, government and the arts, real as they are over time and space, only illustrate the deeper unity of the human condition. From the perspective of a post-Marxian age, however, his argument has a deeper significance.

Millar believed in rank rather than in class: in subordination, as he and his master Adam Smith often called it, rather than in vast and potentially hostile conglomerations like bourgeoisie and proletariat. Such polysyllables figure nowhere in his book. Five years after it appeared, Adam Smith was to introduce a chapter on subordination into his *Wealth of Nations* (V.1), and the debate had already opened in Scotland with Adam Ferguson, a professor of philosophy at Edinburgh and another Whig, when he published his *Essay on the History of Civil Society* in 1767. David Hume disapproved of the book, but he generously reported from London that it was widely admired there; and the poet Gray called it eloquent. Like Millar's after it, Ferguson's book was promptly translated into German and, rather more tardily, into French. Scotland led Europe, in that age, in social studies: anthropology and sociology together, to speak anachronistically, since these three books of 1767-76 – Ferguson, Millar and Adam Smith – are about ancient, medieval and modern history all in one, at once comparative and analytical, factual and theoretical, and in the nature of things they do not recognise any bound or limit between anthropology and its unborn rival.

Nor do they engage in the modern debate about social class, for the simple and easily forgivable reason that they have not heard of it. The sociology of the Scottish Enlightenment was about the subordination of ranks – the factors that cause such subordination and cause it to change. That establishes the point that it is (or was) possible to take an intelligent and even a theoretical interest in social difference without being interested in class at all, as Marx was to understand the term. The theory of rank represents as large a gap as any there is between the socialist world of thought that arose in the 1840s and the preceding age of Enlightenment.

Rank differs from class in more ways than one.[1] It is various – perhaps infinitely various – representing society as something like a pyramid with many steps; whereas class implies, or came to imply, no more than two or three vast groups culminating, in its extreme Marxist version, in class struggle and social civil war. There are other divergences. Rank was (and is) a popular and essentially non-theoretical view of social difference, in the sense that the uneducated can readily believe in it or take it for granted, as the scenes before Agincourt in Shakespeare's *Henry V* vividly illustrate; whereas class was first and last a doctrine for intellectuals. Rank, again, is subtler than class in the sense of admitting more than one defining factor – birth and property, according to Adam Smith, and above all status – whereas class tends to represent an emerging struggle between rich and poor, with the poor as the agents of change.

The contrast between the two competing theories of society, then, is highly paradoxical. One expects intellectuals to hold complex views, on the whole, the uneducated to hold simple ones; and no doubt class theories can be made to look complicated, especially if they are dignified with the

---

1. See Asa Briggs, "The language of 'class' in early nineteenth-century England" (1960), reprinted in his *Collected Essays* vol I, pp. 3-33

jargon of Hegelian dialectic and fitted out with polysyllabic talk about
consciousness and reification. But the real effect of class when it began to
replace rank during and after the Napoleonic wars, in the writings of Saint-
Simon and Marx, was not to subtilise but to simplify. An ignorant by-
stander in daily usage who silently identifies a stranger's probable rank
by dress, gesture and accent, for example, is performing an act of
identification far subtler than the historian who concludes that the Spanish
Civil War was ultimately a struggle between a bourgeoisie and a proletariat.
The real charm of class, one sometimes feels, to the intellectual mind of
the nineteenth and early twentieth centuries, was that it was easy and
portable, 'For most Marxists', as F.R. Leavis perceptively remarked in *For
Continuity* (1933), 'the attraction of Marxism is simplicity'. Intellectuals may
sometimes like things to look complicated. But they can also like them to be
simple. The most seductive combination, one suspects, would be to look com-
plicated and be simple at the same time.

For all these reasons the interest of Millar's argument of 1771 has been
largely obscured: not because it is obscure in itself, which it never is, but
because in terms of the wider argument he could not see, or be expected to
see, where the issue now lies. In accepting or assuming the theory of rank, the
Enlightenment was not to know that a counter-theory was about to be born.
That leaves their writings looking a trifle bland; nor would their views
about prehistory, by now, excite the respect of any living scholar. Millar
had 'no prejudices of veneration in his character', as Francis Jeffrey wrote of
him after his death, hinting at radicalism; but he was not an original theorist
and did not claim to be one. Oddly enough something similar, in a mildly
qualified form, could be said of Marx and his theory of class. It is strange
that this should have been overlooked, since he was a pedantic German
and one conscientious in naming his sources. His theory of class was never,
strictly speaking, expounded in its final form, since it belongs to those
portions of *Das Kapital* left incomplete at his death in 1883; but enough
has survived to make his position clear, and it is confirmed by a highly
important letter of March 1852 where he openly denied having discovered
either the theory of class or the class war – his contribution having been to
show how classes are linked to phases of productive development, and
how the coming class war must inevitably lead to a dictatorship of the
proletariat.[1] Since there have been no such class wars in industrial states,
the second proposition has not exactly worn well, and the first is persuasive
only by means of highly elaborate interpretation. Like others one can easily

---

1. 'No credit is due to me for discovering the existence of classes in modern society or
the struggle between them. Long before me bourgeois historians had described
the historical development of the class struggle, and bourgeois economists the
economic anatomy of the classes' (Marx to Georg Weydemeyer, 5 March 1852)

think of, Marx was mostly unoriginal when he was right and original when he was wrong. What matters, for the moment, is that he should have been wholly aware that the theory of class was in no way his invention.

The Enlightenment view of social difference had this in common with such nineteenth-century views as Saint-Simon's and Marx's, that it was first and last a theory of history. Millar's book, for example, like Rousseau's second *Discours* (1754) before it, treats prehistory and the first creation of settled societies. But history here points in opposite directions. For Montesquieu and his followers it had illustrated the constancy-in-flux of human nature; for Saint-Simon and Marx, its profound inconstancy. Consciousness itself, as Marx believed, had been profoundly changed both by feudalism and by the industrial revolution, and socialism would soon change it again; man is not now what he was, and he is about to become another thing. That argument between the humanism of the Enlightenment and the relativism of its successors will not easily be settled, but the collapse of communism might be said to have left the game drawn, for the moment, in the humanist's favour, in that a free market in eastern Europe may imply that consciousness was not, after all, profoundly and permanently altered by socialism, that a human instinct for individual self-advancement can survive even three-quarters of a century of deep-freeze submersion. Or perhaps it is too soon to say. In a sense it will always be too soon to say, since a question as vast as that cannot be settled by a single instance or set of instances. Montesquieu's contention that the diversity of nations and races only serves to underline an ultimate consistency, much like a variation in music, is in any case so interpretable that the argument cannot just stop there, and it is bound to continue. The humanistic backlash of recent years is none the less notable, however, after a century and more of dogmatic relativism in the fashion of Marx, Nietzsche and Freud; in *Beast and Man* (1978), for example, Mary Midgley has persuasively argued as a philosopher that anthropologists and sociologists in recent times have tended to see only differences because differences were all they were looking for, so that the humanistic doctrine of the unchanging human heart may, in the end, be less absurd than we have recently been encouraged to suppose.

There are other contrasts here. Though Millar had read travel-books and even fleetingly mentions the Congo, neither he nor his master Montesquieu, in an age before archaeology and anthropological field work were born, show much profound acquaintance with evidence beyond the textual or with worlds beyond the classic ages of Greece and Rome and the intervening epoch of European feudalism. As seen from the present, their evidence is thin. Marx too was a classicist by education, but his range was wider, especially in his later years when, as his ethnological notebooks show, he took a passionate interest in Third World topics (as they would now be called) like American Indians, and more than his modern admirers have cared to acknowledge in theories of race. These speculations, like those of Engels concerning primitive communism, are not now much respected by anthropologists, being based on fanciful and largely discredited sources on prehistory like the American ethnologist Lewis Morgan; but for good or ill they make the Marxist mix richer, historically and geographically, than the Enlightenment. The European vision broadened enormously in the nineteenth century, by exploration and settlement. Whether that was to the ultimate advantage or disadvantage of what Marx and Engels wrote is another matter.

The most provocative contrast, however, between the two traditions lies nowhere here, but in the simple fact that the luminaries of the Enlightenment saw wealth rather than poverty as an agent for change, and change for the better. They wrote like Whig magnates.

Since the world, with the death of socialism, is returning by leaps and bounds to that opinion, the Enlightenment view now possesses an interest beyond the merely curious. Four years before Millar, Adam Ferguson in his *Essay* had considered the subordination of ranks required of any settled and peaceful society as necessarily based on an earlier accumulation of private wealth. Such wealth, he believed, was utterly essential to the civilising task of turning brutal warlords into the rulers of settled and prosperous states, and must precede it:

Before this important change is admitted, we must be accustomed to the distinction of ranks; and before they are sensible that subordination is requisite, they must have arrived at unequal conditions by chance (p. 152).

In other words, the highly desirable goal of a settled society can only be based on an existing ownership of property, where some have more and others have less or none; so that political power in peaceful states, as under the Whig constitution of 1689, is likely to be an effect rather than a cause of unequal ownership. The doctrine of the economic base is already here; and Montesquieu had already hinted at it, though not as a universal law.[1] Ferguson was quite clear, like Millar after him, that social and economic institutions commonly underlie political change and promote such change. His chief emphasis lay on the institution of justice – statutes, judges, law courts and the like – which, as in Adam Smith, presuppose private property and largely exist to guarantee property. Property comes first; and only societies where there are rich as well as poor, in that view, can sustain

---

1. Cf. *L'Esprit des Lois* xviii.22, on hereditary rights in the early Middle Ages: 'La disposition de la loi civile força la loi politique.'

forms of justice, civil liberties and the civilised arts, so that inequality of condition is in no sense a matter for regret. In fact it is out of property, and the laws that protect it, that liberty is born. Liberty, he wrote candidly, 'appears to be the portion of polished nations alone' (p. 401); a non-reversible proposition, one may be sure, since Ferguson must have been aware that France in 1767 was polished but not free.

This is an arresting argument to generations like our own now emerging from the easy assumption that private wealth is socially conservative in its effects. Ferguson and Millar believed the reverse; so did Adam Smith. Liberty, in their view, and the very search for liberty, needs rich men, and not a few of them; and since not everybody can be rich, one may say that liberty needs inequality of condition in order to seek and achieve equality before the law. The less there is of one equality, they might have agreed, the more there is likely to be of the other. Political advance arises out of inequality, they believed; and Orwell's contention in *Animal Farm* that equality of condition, or rather the search for it, naturally leads to despotism is one they would no doubt have been happy to endorse. Like the ancient historians he had read, Millar was of course aware that wealth can corrupt. None the less it can lead naturally to demands for civil rights by the rich against their rulers, whether Stuart or Bourbon; and it can sometimes lead, as after 1689, to liberty itself. 'The farther a nation advances in opulence and refinement', Millar wrote in his fourth chapter, echoing Ferguson's point about polished nations,

> it has occasion to employ a greater number of merchants, of trades-
> men and artificers; and as the lower people, in general, become
> thereby more independent in their circumstances, they begin to exert
> those sentiments of liberty which are natural to the mind of man,
> and which necessity alone is able to subdue (p. 185).

So the most natural effect of wealth, though not an inevitable effect, is political radicalism: a limited monarchy, for example, as opposed to tyranny, perhaps even a republic, and extensions of the suffrage. Just as poverty tends to acquiesce in despotism, as in slave states, so private wealth tends to be radical, in that view, obliterating memories of a 'former state of servitude', enfeebling traditional authority by creating a sense of independence, and weakening hereditary influences. Wealth in that case is a necessary, though not a sufficient, cause of progress. 'Money becomes more and more the only means of procuring honours and dignities' (p. 187), Millar remarks without regret, as if the prospect of California were nothing much to worry about.

The worry about new wealth only began when it started to happen. Some thirty years later William Wordsworth, by then an ex-revolutionary, complained in his sonnet "O Friend!" (1802) that

The wealthiest man among us is the best,

as if this were a shocking infringement on the status of old families. Jane

Austen's novels can be deprecating about the social pretensions of the
newly rich who try to ignore their origins. It is easy to forget that
conservative interests were once fiercely critical of competitive wealth-
creation and the commercial spirit, and for good reason. Commerce was
radical. Charles Dickens, as a radical, profoundly admired the active
commercial spirit – Daniel Doyce, the lively engineer-inventor in *Little
Dorrit*, illustrates the point – and no one has ever shown what, in its social
effects, is likely to be conservative about economic competition. By the early
years of the nineteenth century Wordsworth found the commercial spirit
dreadfully vulgar, which perhaps at times it is. Ferguson, Millar and Adam
Smith saw it as the engine of civilisation as well as of social change, which it
surely can be, and it is an argument worth reviving. As Yeltsin's Russia may
yet show, there is no economic system more likely to allow the poor and the
unconnected to rise and threaten a hereditary caste or privileged
nomenklatura than a competitive one. New wealth threatens old far more
dangerously than socialism ever did; and while established interests like a
monarchy or the Soviet Communist Party hardly need private wealth at all,
being endowed with the privileges of state, any radical who tries to subvert
such systems will need wealth; he will need to be rich himself, that is, if he is
to create and promote an effective radical opposition, or to enlist, as Lenin
and Hitler once did, the support of those who are. The sobering truth is
that radicals and revolutionaries need private riches more than their rulers.

It is now time to return to Christopher Hill, that Marxist survivor in an age of
disillusion. Like E.P. Thompson, he left the British Communist Party in 1956-
7 in protest against the Soviet invasion of Hungary, and his independent cre-
dentials have been unassailed for a generation or more. But independent
Marxism, too, is now under threat, and with reason. To consider again the
terms of his 1991 article in *History Today*, Hill argued there that what 1989
demonstrated was not the death of Marxism but of the communist parties. It
probably signalled both, but the death of an abstraction is admittedly harder to
certify than that of a person or party, and it will take more than an Enlightenment
Scot like John Millar, or even Montesquieu, to overturn his case. But then that
is less because it is strong than because, in certain important respects, it is
simply nebulous. Consider this passage from Hill's "Premature obsequies?":

> During the past century many Marxist ideas have been incorporated
> into the thinking of historians, including those who regard themselves
> as anti-Marxists. That society must be seen as a whole; that politics,
> the constitution, religion and literature are . . . related to the economic
> structure and development of that society; that there are ruling
> classes; all these are now commonplace.

The trouble is that they were commonplace two centuries ago and before

Marx was born. They were known to anyone who had read Montesquieu, Ferguson, Millar or Adam Smith, and not all of them were wholly unfamiliar to Aristotle, Hobbes and Locke before them. Christopher Hill simply has not read enough if he imagines that Marx was the first to see society as a whole – Macaulay did that in his famous third chapter of his *History of England,* which appeared in 1849, the very year Marx settled in England – or that Marx invented the concept of a ruling class, or that he was the first to link political and artistic advances to the economy. Marx neither invented the doctrine of the economic base nor claimed to have done so. He profoundly admired Aristotle, who perhaps did, and in *Das Kapital* he quotes Montesquieu, Ferguson and Adam Smith, though not (as it happens) Millar; and in his eighth chapter he discusses Macaulay's third chapter, though without approbation.

A lack of reading may seem an impertinent charge to make against scholars, but that is to misunderstand the direction in which lives are lived. Even scholars, after all, often form their dogmatic opinions, sometimes for life, before they have read a word of the matter, and later reading can be partial and omissive. In 1978, in the foreword to *The Poverty of Theory,* E.P. Thompson confessed that he 'commenced to reason' in his thirty-third year, which suggests that his first dozen years and more as a Marxist activist were lived in a spirit of blind obedience. Moses Finley, an ancient historian, once explained in an interview that his lifelong dedication to Marxism began as a freshman in a New York college at the age of eighteen when, after listening to some boring classes, he heard Marx expounded in what proved to be, for him, an irreversible revelation. At that time he had not so much as heard of Marx; so it is possible for highly intelligent beings to be converted, and permanently converted, by authors of whom they have read nothing. In 1983, in one of his last books, *Politics in the Ancient World,* Finley rightly deplored the vulgar habit of calling all class analysis Marxist, since (as he said) it is in fact at least as old as Aristotle. Not everyone is so informed and scrupulous. A German professor of similar sympathies once told me it would be quite wrong to imply he was unacquainted with the writings of Marx and Engels, since he had read the *Communist Manifesto* more than once. The *Manifesto* is a pamphlet, not a book, and Marx and Engels were voluminous authors; but he plainly thought that a sufficient answer. Marxists were not just ignorant of the world. They were ignorant of Marx.

It may seem strange that so many modern historians should be content to talk as if social theory were an innovation of the 1840s. But there may be an explanation. Aristotle, when he spoke of the struggle between rich and poor, was making the deeply anti-democratic point that the poor only want democracy in order to expropriate the rich; and the Scottish

Enlightenment, for its own high-minded reasons, was also actively in favour of inequality and private wealth. These are arguments that have not usually recommended themselves to historians in a democratic and even egalitarian age. Victorian socialism did not deny its intellectual origins, and Marx's debt to Aristotle was one he often acknowledged. In fact he was proud of it. The twentieth century has usually preferred to ignore his sources, both ancient and modern, though H.M. Hyndman in an admiring autobiography openly hailed him as the Aristotle of the nineteenth century. Idolised for decades behind a wall of barbed wire, and venerated for even longer by earnest spirits outside the Wall, his footnotes were neglected and his sources unread. Those sources were often anti-popular, openly favourable to the rich, and ignorant of the new conditions soon to be created by an industrial revolution. No wonder, then, if the Enlightenment, which candidly believed in private wealth as an agent of progress, was simply written out of the script after Marx's death![1]

There is a danger of creating and perpetuating a large myth of intellectual history, by now, if assertions that Marx invented the theory of class or the idea of the economic base are allowed to pass unremarked; and the academia of the English-speaking world may soon come to look like a sort of Masada or last redoubt of impenitent Marxism. 'Jack Hexter is the doyen of anti-Marxists', Christopher Hill writes triumphantly, 'but when he tells us that Shakespeare's *Richard II* is about property . . . his approach is manifestly Marxist'. But is it? There is a river in Macedon, as a Welshman says in another of Shakespeare's plays, and a river in Monmouth, and one does not need to be a Marxist to be interested in property. In his *Politics* Aristotle insisted that it is a merely accidental feature of oligarchies to be ruled by a few, of democracies to be ruled by the many. His base was already economic: 'the real point of difference is poverty and wealth' (1276b). So perhaps J.H. Hexter is an Aristotelian, though I suspect he is better left to speak for himself.

Or perhaps both Hill and Hexter are Millarists, and should both be invited to read his book and tell us. More than two centuries ago Millar believed that property defined power and directed where it would go, and his theory of rank has worn far better than any theory of class. If we could make the invisible Scot visible again, along with his sources among the *philosophes* and his Scottish contemporaries, we might liberate ourselves from more than the tyranny of communism that Hill, like others, discovered forty years too late. We might liberate ourselves from an obsession with class.

---

1. Or only a little earlier. Cf. W.G. Runciman in *Social Science and Political Theory* who, after discussing Aristotle and Montesquieu, insists that Saint-Simon in the early years of the nineteenth century was 'the first to see . . . that the economic structure of society is in some sense the basis for the form of the State' (p. 27)

3
The Idea of Conservative Revolution

By the late twentieth century the intellectual fashion for revolution may have had its day. It was once thought the modern age had been made by it; but sustained stability now looks more interesting, since stable societies are not just more comfortable but at times more radical too. That was not always plain. 'I suppose what connotes a revolution is shots', William Gerhardie once remarked gaily, as a refugee from Bolshevism. 'They have a way of conveying a sense of importance'. It is that sense of revolutionary importance, or self-importance, that has dramatically faded in recent years. A word has lost its radical chic. Why, it is now asked, were revolutions ever supposed by nature to be radical? And why, in any case, should societies not change faster and more efficiently without them?

The surprising truth, now difficult to recover, is that revolution has not always been thought of in radical terms at all. That use of the term was exceptional before the nineteenth century. The word was once conservative. That this should be thought odd looks even odder when one reflects that many revolutions even in recent times, like the Iranian, have been manifestly conservative in effect, in intent, and even in both; so that it is now hard to resist the conclusion that recent theories of revolution have been seriously out of touch with reality, and doubly out of touch with such far-from-radical events as the English Revolution of 1689. What has recently been gained is an appreciation of stability – of what it can achieve in the way of social change, since few societies change as fast as those that are predictably stable. That means recovering, in a new age, a discarded sense of conservative revolution.

Most modern theorists have assumed revolution to be indissolubly linked to radical ideology, transforming political systems in favour of the poor by a deliberate and pre-announced design. In that familiar model, intellectual élites like Jacobins or Bolsheviks demand social change; the demand is violently acted on; and societies change, for the better, as an effect of a violent act – a sort of word-made-flesh. As a general account, however, all that looks increasingly hard to swallow. For one thing, societies are inclined to change of themselves, and without their rulers – revolutionary or otherwise – intending them to do so. In the modern age, at least, it is the stationary state that is exceptional; for good or ill change is natural to human societies, especially in industrial states; so that intellectuals do not need to write or speak, or rulers to act, to make it happen, though they may often have to act to prevent it or to moderate it. Again, rulers who seize power through revolution may hold much the same views about the social order as those they replace. Above all, changes deliberately wrought by governments are highly unreliable in achieving what they were meant to achieve. Politics is a world of unintended effects, and the twentieth century is littered with instances of counter-effective revolutions, so to speak: seizures of power designed or supposed to be popular that have ended by entrenching the privileges of a ruling caste. The Soviet system that collapsed in 1989 is one notorious instance among many. There can be no easy assumption in public affairs that intent, real or imagined, equals effect.

Modern theorists of revolution are still inclined to talk as if nothing like that ever happened. 'Revolution is a form of change within a social system', wrote Chalmers Johnson in 1964, in *Revolution and the Social System*, as if remarking on something uncontroversial. In the following year Michael Walzer, in a study of Calvinism called *The Revolution of the Saints*, confidently associated revolution with radical ideology, as if no conservative in history had ever made one. In 1972 John M. Dunn echoed those assumptions in *Modern Revolutions*, where he called revolution 'a form of massive, violent and rapid social change' that tries to 'embody a set of values in a new, or at least renovated, social order'. Much of that harked back to Hannah Arendt's influential study *On Revolution* in 1963, where, after the briefest of acknowledgements to conservative revolution as a notion long since obsolete, she openly based her generalisations on the three most famous revolutions, after the English, in modern history: the American, the French, and the Russian. But no convincing reason has ever been offered to show that 1776, 1789 and 1917 were representative of revolutions in general; and the very fact that they are famous, influential and heavily mythologised might lead one to suspect the reverse.

The sober truth is that modern theories of revolution by now fail to account for many, and perhaps most, of the instances. The theory of revolution is a fantasy of revolution. Consider South America, a continent rife with political violence throughout the century. In the classic case power was seized, always with force and usually with bloodshed, by an officer whose chief concern was self-promotion. Colonels like to be generals, it is said, and revolution can be a way to do it. Modern theorists are helpless to describe such events, commonplace as they are, since they are eager to ignore the simple truth that new rulers can easily hold the same notions about the social order as those they violently replaced; and they can be reluctant to accept that revolution may involve no social change of any kind, whether massive and radical or trivial and slow. Shakespeare's Macbeth murdered Duncan to take power. He then used his kingship in a dishonourable way, but there is no hint in the play that he held a theory of

government or social order different from the murdered king's; still less
that he instituted, or sought to institute, social change. If revolution means
the violent seizure of power in a state, then it is often socially neutral and
sometimes socially regressive. What is radical about revolution?

It is by now so widely believed that revolutions are ideological that it
demands a large effort of will to recall that for most of modern history
they have had no connection with any theory of government whatever,
beyond the simple, unimpeachable notion that rulers rule. Composing *The
Prince* in 1513, Machiavelli showed strikingly little interest in whether
his ideal ruler would share or fail to share the assumptions of his rivals
about what power is for. The ruler has power, he implied, because he
wants it; to be violently succeeded, unless he is ruthless and flexible
enough, by some one who wants it as much and knows better how to get it
and hold it. In twentieth-century terms, Machiavelli's sense of revolution
might be called South-American, and it is a reasonable guess that most
twentieth-century revolutions have been more or less in that style. Others,
like events in Ireland after 1916 or in Iran since 1979, have been arguably
ideological, but in frankly conservative ways.

'The object of Revolution', Lord Acton once wrote in his notes,
equivocating elegantly on the double sense of the word, 'is the prevention
of revolution'. People sometimes seize power to prevent change. Radical
revolution, by contrast, is a rather recent idea, and it is only as late as the
nineteenth century that the word became securely a part of the stock-in-trade
of advanced opinion. That new usage was to have its amusing side-effects.
The exiled Kerensky, for example, was fond of denying that the events of
October-November 1917 that threw him from power in Russia deserved
to be called a revolution at all, resentful of the radical dignity the word
might confer on the Bolsheviks. He preferred to call it a *putsch*. His successful
rival Lenin agreed with him, at least as to the dignity of the word: Arthur
Ransome tells in his *Autobiography* of 1978 how Lenin cheerfully remarked
to him, in the early months of 1918, that the October Revolution had
already outlived the seventy days of the Paris Commune of 1871 'and was
now fairly to be called a revolution and not a revolt'. That was evidently to
stake a claim to historical dignity. The claim that Hitler made a revolution in
Germany after January 1933 was one commonly made by the friends, not the
enemies, of National Socialism; since 1945 German historians have usually
preferred to call January 1933 a *Machtergreifung* or seizure of power, as
if conscious that to call it the Nazi Revolution might appear to justify it.

All this amounts to a myth of virtue: by the early twentieth century
revolutions tended to look virtuous, at least in intent. In Marxist circles,
where Victorian assumptions were apt to flourish uncritically after they
had lost their force elsewhere, revolution was commonly supposed to

signify a shift from one social system to a better. 'All revolutions',
Christopher Hill has written, are 'caused by the breakdown of the old
society',[1] as if the ambitions of politicians are never paramount in human
affairs. Superstitions of progress linger on. The central issue of revolution
'is in the last resort a simple one: do human social conditions have to be
as unequal and as unjust as everywhere they now are?'[2] But it has still to
be explained why equality would be any more just than inequality, or why
change is likely to be for the better, or why a revolutionary should be
interested in social change at all. The apostles of revolution have issued a
blank cheque of an argument, unsigned and unwarranted.

The sources of the word may help to explain how these multiple confusions
arose.[3] As a term of European politics, 'revolution' is late medieval,
'revoluzione' being recorded in Italian as early as the 1350s to describe
violent political change, and by the sixteenth century Florentine historians
were using it to describe seizures of power by the Medicis or their
opponents. Machiavelli was not notably fond of the word, being more at
home with such studiously neutral terms as 'mutazione di stato'; and in
English the word is first recorded in a political sense no earlier than 1600,
in a translation from the Italian. It was hardly an Elizabethan political
term, then: but it had already been used by Montaigne in his *Essais* (II.xii,
III.xiii) in a political way and in texts available to the Elizabethans.
Shakespeare used it only four times in his plays, and in senses never clearly
political; on the other hand his 59th sonnet suggests that such a usage
might not have seemed wholly strange to him, at least as an instance of a
larger law of nature, the law of cyclical change:
>   Whether we are mended, or whe'er better they,
>   Or whether revolution be the same,
hinting at the metaphor of a heavenly body returning to its starting-point,
or to the full turn of a wheel. Revolution is what keeps things as they are,
and a metaphor that alludes to Fortune's wheel can as readily be applied to
dynastic change. As Fortune governs men's lives, so do affairs of state
tend to return to where they began. *Plus ça change*. . . . For the European
Renaissance, political revolution was fundamentally and effortlessly
preservative, and conservative revolution was not a paradox but a self-
evident association of ideas.
    It was natural, then, for Clarendon to call the restoration of Charles II

1. Christopher Hill, "A bourgeois revolution" in *Three British Revolutions 1641,
    1688, 1776*, p. 111
2. J.M. Dunn, *Modern Revolutions*, p. 1
3. See Arthur Hatto, "Revolution", in *Mind 58* (1949); J.M. Goulemot, "Le mot
    révolution", in *Annales historiques de la Révolution Française 39* (1967)

in 1660 a revolution or 'full compassing' in his *History of the Rebellion*
(XI.200); as a royalist, he naturally saw himself as a revolutionary. The
wheel of English fortune had passed from kingship to the base, impious
tyranny of the Cromwellians and back to a legitimate heir; so that the .
events of 1642-9 were not a revolution but a rebellion. Nobody is known
to have called the English Civil War a revolution at the time, though the
word is occasionally used in the plural as if to acknowledge that the seizure
of power by Parliament belonged to that wider class of events.[1] It was only as
late as the nineteenth century that it became at all common to call it a
revolution, and that usage was French before it was English. Even John
Locke in the 1680s does not seem to think that Cromwell and Pym were
revolutionaries, and seventeenth-century Englishmen of whatever loyalty
knew the war between king and parliament by such uneasy phrases as 'the
late troubled times', 'the troubles', 'distractions', 'intestine broils', 'bloody
and unnatural wars' and the like; none of them suggestive of enthusiasm.

At this great distance, for all that, there is a clear case for calling the
English Civil War a revolution, and the phrase 'the English Revolution' is
by now enshrined in the titles of learned works. A difficulty, however, remains.
How can one reasonably attribute to the war of 1642-9 enactments completed
before it began? It was in 1628, after all, that Parliament had enacted that the
King's will could not override *habeas corpus*; in 1641 that the Long Parliament
abolished Star Chamber and its ecclesiastical counterpart High Commission,
effecting a large measure of freedom of the press. The Grand Remonstrance
of 1641, months before war began, speaks with pride of these achievements,
and of bringing wicked advisers to justice; and it was not a civil war that had
done it. It seems odd to refer to parliamentary enactments, however sweeping,
as a revolution. The rights of Englishmen had been restored before the
Civil War began, and it is not plain that they achieved rights by that war
not statutorily possessed before 1642. That makes it harder to see the civil
war as ameliorative, as modern theories of revolution demand. When
Guizot began to publish his *Histoire de la révolution d'Angleterre* in 1826
he was plainly drawing the Cromwellians into the long shadow of the Jacobins;
and as a Frenchman he was not to know that the shadow of the French
Revolution obscured a remote constitutional struggle in early Stuart England.
Which was the first revolution, then, to be widely hailed by that name at
the time?

---

1. For example, in Anthony Ascham's *Of the Confusions and Revolutions of
   Government*; William Sancroft's *Modern Politics* of 1652, an anonymous
   royalist pamphlet by the future Archbishop of Canterbury who writes in veiled
   scorn of 'alterations and revolutions in kingdoms' (sig. E2) and of 'a general
   innovation' caused by 'state-novelists', meaning the Cromwellians.

The answer is likely to be the English Revolution of 1688-9, the Glorious Revolution by which James II was forced into exile and Parliament proclaimed his daughter Mary and her husband, William of Orange, joint monarchs: events hailed as revolutionary as they occurred. 'The Popists in office lay down their commissions and fly', wrote John Evelyn in his diary on 2nd December 1688, a few days before James II left London for France. 'Universal consternation among them: it looks like a revolution.' Whether Evelyn uses the word here in its preservative sense is not clear. He may have meant something as severely neutral as a violent change from ruler to ruler, and no more; or he may have seen it, as many did, as a full compassing and a restoration of ancient rights.

Locke is as indecipherable here as Evelyn. He returned to England from his Dutch exile in February 1689, a day or two before Parliament offered William and Mary the crown, when *Two Treatises of Government* was in large part already written. But he extended and revised it under the pressures of events themselves between February and August 1689, publishing it in 1690. The book scarcely uses the word 'revolution' at all, and then only in a severely neutral sense, usually in the plural. For example:

> This slowness and aversion in the people to quit their old constitutions has, in the many revolutions which have been seen in this kingdom, in this and former ages, still kept us to or, after some interval of fruitless attempts, still brought us back again to our old legislative of King, Lords and Commons (II.223).

Shakespeare and Clarendon would have had no difficulty with that. On the probable assumption that 'still' here means 'always', it amounts to an entirely traditional use of 'revolution' as a preservative act.

'Resistance', by contrast, was radical. In Locke it most commonly means the resistance of a people to executive power (e.g. II.203 f.), and hence a rebellion or attempted revolution (II.226 f.) – 'an opposition not to persons but authority'. It is likely enough, then, that though Evelyn and Locke shared the general view of 1689 as a revolution, they also shared the view that it was an act preservative of the ancient rights of Englishmen; and a broadly neutral sense of the word remains in Europe throughout the next century. French historians in the eighteenth century occasionally regard England as a revolutionary model, and William of Orange as the type of revolutionary leader, the classic Machiavellian 'prince' of the eighteenth-century European mind. But all such revolutions are without a social dimension, and nobody imagined William III or his followers purposed any change in the nature of British society.

The Machiavellian model, in short, effortlessly prevails. Men take power because power is what they want and because it is something worth having. The French Academy dictionary of 1762 gives the severely neutral sense of 'changement politique', which is much like what Samuel Johnson had offered as a definition seven years before – 'change in the state of a government or country' – citing William and Mary, in his dictionary, as the instance best known to his countrymen. That neutral sense was fully endorsed by another Tory, David Hume. 'It is seldom', he remarked laconically in *The History of Great Britain* of 1754-6, 'that the people gain anything by revolutions in government'; and the fact that 'violent innovations' some-times improved constitutions, as 1689 exceptionally did, was an oddity of the British case. Even Thomas Paine, as late as 1792, thought something like that, and in his introduction to the second part of *Rights of Man* he called recent events in America and France counter-revolutions, since (unlike real revolutions) they have affected the lives of ordinary people:

> The revolutions which formerly took place in the world had nothing
> in them that interested the bulk of mankind. They extended only to
> a change of persons and methods, and not of principles, and rose
> and fell among the common transactions of the moment. What we
> now behold may not improperly be called a 'counter-revolution'.
> Conquest or tyranny, at some early period, dispossessed man of his
> rights, and he is now recovering them.

For the bulk of mankind, plainly, revolutions commonly keep things as they are. They are not even expected to do otherwise.

The radical sense of revolution, socialist or other, is slow to evolve, and its growth is confused and mysterious.

None more mysterious than its use to describe events in British America between 1775 and 1783. That act of separation was not widely hailed as a revolution at the time on either side of the Atlantic: in that sense it differs strikingly from the English Revolution of 1689. Americans who opposed those events as loyalists preferred to call them a rebellion; most were content to speak of a war or contest. Lafayette, it is true, calls it a revolution in a letter to Washington of 30th December 1777, a year and more after independence had been declared; but the remark was exceptional in the 1770s, and he was not an American. Daniel Leonard, an American Tory writing in 1775, shortly before the Declaration of Independence in *The Origin of the American Contest with Great Britain*, calls it 'the most wan-ton and unnatural rebellion that ever existed' (p. 40). Adam Smith, who delayed the publication of *The Wealth of Nations* to consider these events, calls them uncommittedly in his last pages 'the present disturbances' (V.iii); and the Declaration of July 1776 avoids the word 'revolution' altogether, speaking rather of a need to 'dissolve the political bands' and appealing in classic Enlightenment language to the 'separate and equal station to which the Laws of Nature and of Nature's God entitle them'. Separation is not revolution, and hardly anyone thought it was.

An awkward handful of exceptions still needs to be considered. In a letter of 27th July 1776, weeks after the Declaration, the republican fire-brand Samuel Adams exclaimed: 'Was there ever a revolution brought about, especially so important as this, without great internal tumults and violent convulsions?' But that remark, if carefully pondered, remains consistent with a strictly neutral sense of the word. On 3rd May 1779, again, Richard Henry Lee wrote to his friend Jefferson about 'our glorious revolution', as if eager, against the odds, to make a radical battle-cry out of a conservative term. But revolution was never the usual description of Washington's victory in either country in its own century, merely one possible description among others. There are two patriotic books of the 1780s by David Ramsay of Charleston, for example, that celebrate the term in their very titles: *The History of the Revolution in South-Carolina* (1785) and *The History of the American Revolution* (1789); and on 10th April 1789, three months before the fall of the Bastille, George Washington thanked Crèvecoeur for some books, remarking in a letter that they had shown him a new climate of opinion in France, and used the significant and resounding phrase:

The American Revolution, or the peculiar light of the age, seems to have opened the eyes of almost every nation in Europe, and the spirit of equal liberty appears fast to be gaining ground everywhere.

Considering William III had once been a hero to some historians in colonial America, it is striking how seldom the thirteen colonies refer to the English Revolution of 1689 in order to justify their actions, how seldom they call on the name of William III to vilify George III. The colonial appeal after 1776 is more often to the rights of man than to the rights of Englishmen, approbation of 'our British ancestors' being jumbled with appeals to the Ancients and to the French Enlightenment. It seems likely, then, that the radical sense of 'revolution' was entrenched in American usage no earlier than the 1820s. In 1828 Noah Webster, for example, in his *American Dictionary,* instances the American along with the English and the French, calling revolution 'a material or entire change in the constitution of government', which certainly sounds rather more than a bloody shift from ruler to ruler; and he adds provocatively, at the time of the Greek War of Independence: 'we shall rejoice to hear that the Greeks have effected a revolution'.

To the modest evidence from eighteenth-century America, however, may be added a crumb from home. In 1784 Richard Price, a dissenting minister of Enlightenment views who was shortly to anger Edmund Burke, published a rapturously pro-American pamphlet called *Observations on the Importance of the American Revolution*. He called it a 'revolution in favour of human liberty', as if that were something of a new idea, opening 'a new era in the history of mankind': the most important event in human history since Christianity, and one ultimately destined to benefit Britain as well as America. Radical revolution, then, was a possible paradox on both sides of the Atlantic even before the fall of the Bastille in July 1789. But those who thought so – certain Jeffersonians, a radical Dissenter in London, and George Washington – and the terms in which they thought it, all suggest that the view was new, daring and intellectual. Radical revolution is a late Enlightenment paradox, in that case: the notion of a few advanced spirits as the eighteenth century grew towards its violent close.

The American Revolution, then, sits uneasily inside this story of a word. If the founders of the American Republic were English Whigs, they were strenuously reluctant to say so, though they occasionally acknowledged a debt to a remoter English past. The first United States warship was called the *Alfred*; and in 1777 John Adams was urging his ten-year-old son to study Stuart history down to the Revolution of 1689 with especial care. But recent British history, he wrote in a letter of March 1777, showed 'how completely their government was corrupted'; and the mood of 1776 was an impatient shaking-off of precedent among the supporters of change – an act of purification that often sought to deny the past altogether.

If it is asked why Americans, on the whole, tended to avoid the term 'revolution' before 1800, the most probable explanation may also be the most surprising. Since the word was still mainly preservative in its implications, it may have been natural to them to avoid it on that ground alone. Preservers at heart such men as Washington, Madison and Jefferson may have been; but in the Declaration of 1776 they offered themselves as heralds of a new age – *novus ordo saeculorum* – not as the revivers of an old. Radical rhetoricians of the age, like Paine, may have found revolution still too backward-looking a term to their taste. That may explain why 1776, unlike 1689, had to wait for decades before it chose to call itself unequivocally by that name.

The Enlightenment view of this tangled issue is vital here, and above all, that of the French *philosophes* and of Rousseau.

It is notable how seldom the *philosophes*, anglophile though they often were, mentioned the English Revolution of 1689. That may have been in part because French royal censorship would have forbidden open praise of an act of usurpation like William III's; in part because the *philosophes* inclined as much to benevolent despotism as to parliamentary rule. Their doctrine of government was a wavering one, constitutionally speaking: intent on freedom of thought and humane penal laws, less clear about how such effects might some day be constitutionally guaranteed or gained.

In his *Lettres Anglaises* of 1734, for example, an early work and much his most radical, Voltaire openly praised the English constitution under which he had recently lived, in the ninth letter, as a 'mélange heureux'. It is not from William III, however, that he derived that happy mixture of King, Lords and Commons or the liberties it guaranteed, but from Magna Carta, and Voltaire's admiration for William always remained faintly secretive. In the eighth letter he praised the English revolutionary settlement in slightly veiled terms, calling England the first nation ever to limit the power of kings; and it was a usurper, as he was to write years later in an unpublished epigram, who had given to the world 'the example of the virtues a king should have'.[1] All that stops short of open praise. Montesquieu, again, admired the British system, and had watched debates at Westminster during his English stay in 1729-31; but in his public writings he prudently lays no approving emphasis on the Glorious Revolution; and in 1765 the *Encyclopédie* of Diderot and d'Alembert refers only innocuously to that event under 'revolution', defining the word neutrally, much as the French Academy had recently done: 'a considerable change brought about in the government of a state'. The article is perhaps faintly subversive in its suggestion that James II had fallen because of popery and despotism, having learned those faults abroad as an exile and mainly in France. But if the *philosophes* thought the English Revolution an example to all mankind, then they took some care to leave that commitment obscure.

But then the only revolution ever consistently sought by the Enlightenment was one of mind. Socialism would change all that. Voltaire, for example, had hailed the mood of Europe after the defeat of France in the Seven Years War as promising 'a revolution that will irresistibly come, and which I shall not have the joy of seeing' – his compatriots being lamentably slow, as usual, he remarks in a letter, at everything:

> Enlightenment grows nearer and nearer, leading towards an outburst at the first opportunity, and then there will be a fine old rumpus (*un beau tapage*); the young are lucky indeed, they will see some fine things (2 April 1764).

But whether Voltaire's *beau tapage* means speeches and pamphlets or bloodshed and civil war remains carefully unclear, even in a private letter. These were dangerous thoughts, even among friends. The *philosophes* had no lucid and consistent view, in any case, how an enlightened state was ever to be created and sustained. It might use violence or it might not. Such violence could at best only be the expression of an idea: it was in no way essential to that idea, as in the next century it was to be essential to Marxism. 'The revolution was in the minds of the people', wrote John

---

1. Voltaire, *Complete Works*, lxxxi.338, from the St Petersburg notebooks, probably composed 1735-50

Adams in a famous phrase to Thomas Jefferson in 1815 – the second president of the United States writing to the third. He was referring to the years 1760-5, which (he claimed) had 'enlightened and informed' American opinion about the intentions of the British parliament. That populist notion is plainly original to the Enlightenment: the notion, that is, that political achievement might reflect not just the ambitions of a few but the aspirations of the many. It is an idea that would have greatly puzzled Machiavelli and Shakespeare. It would not have puzzled the *philosophes*. Enlightenment is first and last an idea: so much so, that it remains eternally wavering and uncertain in its search for specific constitutional means. How mankind might choose to embody such ideas in action it was often content to leave to men of affairs, and to fate.

To turn from the *philosophes* to Rousseau is to confirm that view. Rousseau seldom writes of revolution, though he is publicly indignant at the spectacle of extremes of wealth and poverty, of power and servitude; and in private, at least, hotly anti-monarchical. In 1762, in the third book of *Emile*, he speaks darkly of all human affairs as transient – not least the monarchies of Europe: 'sujets à des révolutions inévitables' whereby the rich would some day grow poor and monarchs in their turn become subjects. It is a risky footnote, as Rousseau plainly knew, and his language remains secretive and ominous. 'We are approaching a state of crisis', he continues, 'and a century of revolutions', adding guardedly:

> I hold it to be impossible that the great monarchies of Europe can
> last much longer; they have all shone brightly, and whatever does
> that is on the point of decline. My own view of the matter has grounds
> more detailed than the maxim itself: but it would be inappropriate
> to declare them, and anyone can see only too well for himself.

No public acclaim for revolution there, but no comfort for rulers either: only a furtive hint at change.

But then, as in America, a preservative word was not easily to be linked to a radical cause, and for a clearly radical use of 'revolution' one has to wait for that late Enlightenment treatise, William Godwin's *Political Justice*. Written by an Englishman a few years after the French Revolution itself, it claims the event was 'instigated by a horror against tyranny' (IV.ii), as if no sense of revolution but a radical one had ever existed. That vividly suggests how rapidly events in France after 1789 had radicalised the term; and Godwin stands as the pioneer of its modern use in English. *Political Justice* is an anti-revolutionary book, being dedicated to gradual perfectibility and non-violence. But its confident assumption that revolutions are made by the poor and the oppressed, or in their name and on their behalf, makes a new age for the word.

Four years later an unknown young French royalist sheltering in London called the English Civil War 'Cromwell's revolution', arguing spiritedly that the French Revolution of which he was a victim would never have happened at all without the example of the English. The *Essai sur les Révolutions* is Chateaubriand's first book, and a highly confusing one: an untidy comparison of revolutions ancient and modern. But it may be the first work of consequence to call Puritan England a revolutionary state, drawing it into an analogy with recent violent events in France. The young Frenchman thought the English Civil War not only an instance of revolution but a grand cautionary model for the future of mankind. The execution of Charles I in 1649 demonstrated 'how far the Jacobins imitated it' in executing Louis XVI: 'I dare to say that if Charles had not been decapitated in London, Louis would probably not have been guillotined in Paris' (chapter 18).

History is hindsight; and if no Englishman in 1649 thought he was watching a revolution, and few Americans in 1776, it was clear to lonely thinkers of the 1790s like Godwin and Chateaubriand that the disorders of contemporary France required some past events to be recategorised. Cromwell's revolution became that only after the French had imitated it. It is 1789, then, that unbinds revolution from its conservative chains, and the socialists were its heirs. The sense of the word shifted lastingly from Right to Left after the Bastille fell.

But then the sheer possibility of purposeful social change is probably not much older than the European Enlightenment. If Machiavelli and Shakespeare saw no prospect of a radically new social order, that was probably because they could imagine no such thing, and would have thought it absurd to try. Those who murder Julius Caesar in Shakespeare's play go about the streets of Rome shouting 'Liberty! Freedom!'; but the play shows that they fail, and it implies that anyone would. In the end, and on the widest view, nothing changes. Men remain what they are: that is the truth, or supposed truth, that makes all revolutions before the American and the French look like a full compassing. The death of Charles I led to the restoration of his son Charles II – what else could it do? The wheel of fortune cannot leave its axis: it can only revolve. Men may shift their place there, for better or worse; but the wheel stays where it is. 'The only thing that stops God from sending a second flood', wrote Chamfort, who was himself to perish in the Terror, 'is that the first was useless'. The death of Caesar prefigures the death of Charles I, of Louis XVI, of the last of the Tsars. Preservative revolution rests on the classic premiss that nothing ever changes, in the end, because in the end nothing ever can; radical revolution on the highly recent notion that the world can change and must.

The shift of horizon that made socialism possible is still unclear, both in time and space. The Enlightenment is the natural place to point; and whatever cautious admiration it may have felt for the British constitutional settlement of 1689 was, after all, an admiration for something called a revolution. But it is a shift fearfully difficult to chart. Somewhere between 1689 and 1789 Shakespeare's Brutus becomes a hero and not just an heroic failure, and paradise moves from past to future in the mind of western man. It is that sense of an arcadian future realisable by concerted action that makes Paine, Jefferson and Robespierre look in retrospect like the first of their kind, a kind now seemingly perennial: the politically utopian intellectual. He may be thrust at times to those edges of public life haunted by the fanatic and the terrorist, but as a type he will not die.

There have been numberless side-effects to the mysterious shift from conservative to radical revolution. One is that conservatives have long since abandoned revolution as an ideal, forgetful how congenial the outcome can be. No British conservative today believes that he lives in a revolutionary state, though he does; none now mouths the Revolution Principles of 1689. The world has simply forgotten conservative revolution. It is puzzled by the notion that violent change might keep things as they are or were; still more by the notion that it might be designed to do so. That puzzlement is itself puzzling, since we are surrounded by instances, and not only in Ireland and Iran.

What, then, was conservative revolution?

To read Machiavelli, Shakespeare and Clarendon in the light of that question is to challenge modern assumptions about power and to re-examine the nature of political change itself: the sudden, bloody shift from ruler to ruler, from Duncan to Macbeth, and the attendant problems of how power is won, consolidated and maintained. Since Shakespeare was a great historian, and a signal part of the education of those who made the English Revolution of 1689 and the American, I name him here with Machiavelli and Clarendon without reserve. The ten plays he devoted to English history, along with *Macbeth* and the Roman plays, deal analytically with ideas of statecraft that Machiavelli and Clarendon might have endorsed. How should an aspiring ruler like Bolingbroke, Cesare Borgia or Oliver Cromwell seize power in a state; and what grounds or pretexts – the enrichment of family or friends, foreign conquest, the defence of the homeland, or ancestral rights – should he think enough? And having seized power, how should he proceed against the deposed ruler and his heirs? Machiavelli's insistence, which Lenin echoed, on 'killing the sons of Brutus' to ensure the succession is all the more urgent as a moral issue for being severely practical. It is precisely when crime offers a supreme reward like total power, after all, that it tempts the conscience even of the virtuous.

The Machiavellian ruler had *vertù* rather than virtue – effective strength, that is, and the will and flexibility to use it. Shakespeare's Macbeth had both, which is his tragedy: they can so easily conflict, and do. Cromwell had both too, as even his bitter enemy Clarendon acknowledged after his death. *The Prince, Macbeth* and *The History of the Rebellion* are works not usually mentioned in the same breath; and yet they share a common interest in 'policy' rather than policies, in how power is efficiently and cunningly won and held. Some people like power, after all, for itself; and the modern electoral cry 'What are your policies?' is one that few rulers before the nineteenth century would have felt themselves under any obligation to answer or even to ponder.

The largest side-effect of radicalising revolution, perhaps, has been to moralise political life. The Enlightenment was already busy at that task: it is a plain implication of Voltaire's *Letters Anglaises* that a nation has a duty to be tolerant and virtuous as well as stable and efficient in the conduct of its affairs. That must have looked a very new assumption in the France of the 1730s. Popular election rapidly intensifies the moral element, and since the nineteenth century it has laid on rulers an obligation to justify to millions what they propose to do or what they have done. The Victorian social debate left politics looking almost exclusively like a moral drama – perhaps even a melodrama, since it sometimes allowed only for heroes and villains. The melodrama of public life is by now a view wholly commonplace in the western world, encouraged by the mass-media and by two-party systems that actively promote a cops-and-robbers view of public debate; and it is a disability of the moralising climate in which life is now lived that few political theorists can easily admit power to be interesting in itself. The suggestion is felt to smack of indecency. It is more or less taboo.

Perhaps that is to be too easily shocked. Is it possible to doubt that, even in the open and unsecretive world of modern democratic states, there are those who find power fascinating in itself? Or if not power, then office and the trappings of office? The practical difficulties of doubting that are overwhelming: in fact it is hard to see how any political system, slave or free, could be maintained without actors moved by a relish for the parts they play. Though a neutral sense of revolution may be hard to recover, it would at least have the merit of draining the word of some of its moral dignity – a dignity it has seldom merited. Whether an ex-socialist age can prove attentive enough to the arguments of great minds who thought and wrote before revolution was supposed to be radical is yet to be seen.

4
The Tory Tradition of Socialism

It is still widely assumed, even in an ex-socialist age, that socialism was always thought of as left-wing – that it collapsed through a technical fault, rather like a jet that looked good on the drawing-board and survived its first trials, only to crash with a full load. Even sceptics and enemies often assume it began all good intentions; and in an era of socialist obituaries like Noel Annan's *Our Age* or François Furet's *Le Passé d'une Illusion*, and among the countless revelations now emerging in eastern Europe, one seldom hears its intentions questioned. The subtext reads 'We meant well'. Hardly anyone seems ready to admit that if socialism favoured the rich and the privileged, in the event, it may have meant to do so. Its halo is still in place.

I want to ask here how it is that, in defiance of the evidence, the name of socialism still sounds benevolent, and how its openly Tory and reactionary traditions have been so thoroughly forgotten: a paradox all the more remarkable in an age familiar with parties called socialist that openly govern in a conservative way.

The Tory tradition of socialism was once plain in its motives and lucid in its arguments. In the world's first industrial zone, which was western Europe, a new commerce of factories, railways and mines had ruthlessly transformed an ancient landscape at dizzying speed, and capitalism (as some were coming to call it) was naturally seen as radical. Parties called liberal that advocated free trade and the free market were rapidly destroying traditional patterns of life, loosening family ties and threatening morality itself. No wonder if Ruskin and Morris, like the Christian Socialists before them, detested the liberal idea of the division of labour which, as they believed, signified a soul-destroying shift from the benevolent village community to the soulless factory bench. Socialism above all meant a horror of the new age: an age of machines and high finance. It was more than conservative. It was reactionary and nostalgic, and in the long march from status to contract it demanded a return to the familiar and time-honoured world of status.

To make the crisis worse, parties called conservative were seen in that age to offer little or no help. By the mid-century they were tacitly collaborating with the liberals, at least in Britain – conceding the suffrage, abandoning traditional landed interests, and silently accepting that protection had had its day. As Disraeli and Marx both bitterly complained, they had surrendered. It was a largely conservative parliament, after all, that abolished the Corn Laws in 1846; another that introduced the Second Reform Act to extend the suffrage twenty-one years later. Conservative government, Disraeli wrote derisively in 1844 in *Coningsby*, meant Tory men and Whig measures. With the liberal idea conquering even its traditional enemies, socialism looked like an anguished protest against that conquering idea. Of course it was anti-radical. As Bertolt Brecht was one day to remark, as a Soviet supporter: 'Communism is not radical:capitalism is radical'; and if people called conservatives would not stand up for ancient values, so the argument went, then people called socialists must.

All that explains the candid Toryism of much socialist writing in Victorian times and since. When Ruskin published his autobiography *Praeterita* in 1885, he was a socialist of some twenty years standing, and *Unto This Last* would one day inspire Gandhi, who translated it. This is how he began his autobiography:

> I am, and my father was before me, a violent Tory of the old school
> – Walter Scott's school, that is to say, and Homer's. I name these
> two out of the numberless great Tory writers because they were my
> own two masters.

The passage had first appeared some years before, in the tenth letter of *Fors Clavigera* in October 1871; and a little earlier still, in the first letter of January 1871, Ruskin had called himself a 'violent Illiberal' but in no way a conservative, since he wanted to destroy all sorts of newfangled things like the new Houses of Parliament and the new town of Edinburgh. His programme was for a sort of Tory Greenery, 'to keep the fields of England green and her cheeks red', as he put it engagingly, with little girls curtseying and boys doffing their hats to any dignified person that went by, including professors. Socialism meant hierarchy and Back to Basics. 'I am for Lordship', Ruskin had already declared, in a letter to the *Daily Telegraph* (20 December 1865) supporting Governor Eyre's brutal suppression of a negro revolt that year in Jamaica, distancing himself from John Stuart Mill and others who had taken part in a 'fatuous outcry' on behalf of liberated slaves:

> They are for Liberty, and I am for Lordship; they are Mob's men,
> and I am a King's man. . . . I am a 'Conservative', and hope foreverto
> be a Conservative in the deepest sense – a Re-former, not a Deformer.

So socialism could mean conservatism in the deepest sense, a return to antiquity and a protest against the new age of liberated man. Ruskin's point was not lost to future ages. Through Gandhi it reached India; and in the 1945-50 Parliament many British MP's named *Unto This Last* as the political book that had influenced them most. No wonder if both the Bolshevik and Menshevik parties, before the first world war, attracted a strikingly high proportion of gentry: though a mere 1.7 per cent of the population of the Russian empire, 22 per cent of the Bolsheviks belonged to the gentry.[1] Socialism naturally attracted the patrician mind.

Hence its worship of authority. Socialists, as Karl Pearson bluntly wrote in 1887, as an eminent academic campaigner, in *The Moral Basis of Socialism*, now have to 'inculcate that spirit which would give offending against the state short shrift and the nearest lamp-post'. The hanging-and-flogging side of socialism was not a late perversion of the Stalinist era. It was there from the start.

Ruskin's remark about Homer and Scott is worth pondering. They were Tory writers, no doubt, for having extolled the antique virtues of feudal and pre-feudal Europe: ancestral loyalty, community, physical courage, all threatened by the modern cash-nexus. Ramsay MacDonald as a young man once revealed, quite independently of Ruskin, that it was a reading of the Waverley novels along with Scottish history that had 'opened out the great world of national life for me and led me into politics'.[2] Just what Walter Scott himself, that arch-Tory, would have thought of all this socialist admiration can only be guessed at, but the political effects of the Waverley novels are of impressive implications. Bernard Shaw applauded the point. In 1921, in *Ruskin's Politics*, he told a lecture-audience of Ruskinians, to their incredulous amusement, that the true heirs of Ruskin (could they butsee it) were the Bolsheviks who had recently seized power in Russia; andthey only found that hard to believe because Ruskin had called himself a Tory. But

> all Socialists are Tory in that sense. The Tory is a man who believes
> that those who are qualified by nature and training for public work,
> and who are naturally a minority, have to govern the mass of the
> people. That is Toryism. That is also Bolshevism. The Russian
> masses elected a National Assembly: Lenin and the Bolshevists
> ruthlessly shoved it out of the way, and indeed shot it out of the way
> as far as it refused to be shoved (p. 31).

In the same year Richard Tawney, in *The Acquisitive Society*, called for a return to Christian values and traditional morality, and he ended his book with a passionate demand for a revival of religious ideals abandoned and forgotten in the demeaning scuffle for wealth. Socialism meant 'a rule of life, a discipline, a standard and habit of conduct', as he put it: it was a traditionalist doctrine and a protest against the modern world.

A few years later the Hungarian Marxist George Lukàcs took up the praise of the Waverley novels, though in a manner not clearly indebted to Ruskin or Ramsay MacDonald. *The Historical Novel* was written in 1936-

---

1. Richard Pipes, *The Russian Revolution 1899-1919,* p. 364
2. *Review of Reviews* 33 (1906) p. 577

7, and it praised Scott as the sort of Tory who could teach socialists some-
thing essential: he had been 'among those honest Tories in the England of
his time who exonerate nothing in the development of capitalism – who
not only see clearly, but also deeply sympathise with, the unending misery
of the people which the collapse of old England brings in its wake'. Old
England means a land of gentry animated by traditional moral values, and
it was the loss of that secure world that socialists mourned – though not
without reservation – with its sense of community, maypole-dancing and
knowing-your-place. Capitalism, as everyone knows, can make the vulgar
uppity, and Ruskin's *Unto This Last* had been an attack on liberal economists
who had seen man as nothing more than 'a covetous machine' without
social affections and with no more moral sense than the lower animals – a
creature wholly indifferent to tradition and God's laws. Medieval times
may have been far from perfect; there was no doubt a 'Rough Side of the
Middle Ages', as William Morris called one of the chapters in 1893 in
Socialism, a book he wrote late in life with Belfort Bax. But medieval
craft guilds had at least conceded power and status to the work-force and
encouraged a love of craftsmanship, and 'bourgeois historians' had been
far too ready to praise what they glibly supposed to be 'the escape of
modern society from a period of mere rapine and confusion into peace,
order and prosperity', by which Morris means the commercial and indust-
rial society that Macaulay and others had once welcomed. He denied that
he was a general apologist for the Middle Ages 'except in relation to modern
times', which perhaps implies that he saw all human history since the
Ancients as a regression. H.M. Hyndman too began his *Historical Basis
of Socialism in England*, in the same year, with an assertion he offered as
uncontroversial: that the labouring masses in the fifteenth century had
enjoyed 'rough plenty', the late Middle Ages being, by common consent,
a period when men and women who worked with their hands were better
off than at any time before or since. Parliamentary government was an
utter failure that should be replaced at once by state rule. Modern times
were the worst of times, and socialists demanded a return.

The return would be to medieval affluence, as they imagined it, and to
traditional family values. In 1845, in *The Condition of the Working Classes
in England*, Engels had expressed horror at the destruction of married life
in the industrial north of England, where he lived: it was plainly
demoralising for women to go out to work, he argued, especially when
the husband was left unemployed at home 'to look after the children and
to do the cleaning and cooking'. Gender-reversal had no charms for the
early socialists.

In Manchester alone there are many hundreds of men who are
condemned to perform household duties. One may well imagine

the righteous indignation of the workers at being virtually turned
into eunuchs. Family relationships are reversed (chapter 7),
the husband being deprived of his manhood, Engels argues indignantly,
and the wife of her womanly qualities; and he hints darkly at sexual liberties
in factories where the employer was rumoured to exercise a *ius primae
noctis* over young women: 'his factory is also his harem'. Hyndman was
to echo the point half a century later in his *Historical Basis*, which revealed
a lively horror of divorce and prostitution and demanded a return to family
life; and as late as 1956 Tony Crosland, in *The Future of Socialism*,
applauded Beatrice Webb for withholding support from the Soviet Union
until it had enacted an anti-abortion law. No doubt they would have
endorsed Marx's hostility to divorce too.

That call was a familiar part of the socialist critique of modern life.
Louis Blanc, for example, in a passionate little pamphlet of 1848 called
Le Socialisme, a reply to Thiers, saw socialism as a stabilising force after
a disruptive half-century and more of revolutions in France, concluding
that the family offered the best model of social perfection, since it illustrated
not individualism but solidarity of interest. The repellent radicalism of
free enterprise was a common complaint among socialists. Capitalism
shocked not because it was old but because it was new. Communism, by
contrast, as Karl Kautsky argued in 1897 in *Communism in Central Europe
in the Time of the Reformation*, dated from 'the childhood of the race'. It
is high finance and the stockmarket that are upstarts, and his book celebrates
pious Christian sects like the Bohemian Brethren of the late Middle Ages
and sixteenth-century Anabaptists, who despised private wealth. It was
only in the sixteenth century, Kautsky argued, that the modern state arose,
and with it a deprived proletariat. After a capitalistic gap of three centuries,
socialism was a rebirth: a revival, not an innovation.

Twentieth-century socialists, too, loved the antique, and it was some-
thing remarked on by their enemies as well as their friends. Maynard
Keynes used to deride Marxists between the two world wars as hopelessly
old-fashioned theorists, but the veneration of Marx is only a particular
instance of a wider tendency to look back. In his late writings on kinship,
for example, based on notes that Marx left at his death in 1883, Engels
had called for a return to prehistoric communism without private property,
an era no longer credited by prehistorians or anthropologists; and the British
anthropologist V. Gordon Childe looked for the natural state of man as far
back as neolithic times, when agriculture (as he believed) was non-competitive
and cooperative. Since Childe's death in 1957 Ken Livingstone, the Marxist
leader of the Greater London Council in the 1970s, has gone one better.
Utopia, he told John Carvel in *Citizen Ken*, belongs to an age antecedent
even to the neolithic: the palaeolithic, when nomadic tribes wandered the

earth as hunter-gatherers 'operating overwhelmingly in a cooperative way'.
There seems to have been no natural limit to socialist nostalgia. Modern
finance, said Livingstone, is an abomination, and one radically unnatural
to man. 'The hunter-gatherer is what humanity is.'

Whether medieval, neolithic or palaeolithic, socialism was from its ori-
gins a hierarchical doctrine, and it habitually venerated aristocracy and
leadership. 'My continual aim', Ruskin wrote in *Unto This Last*,

> has been to show the eternal superiority of some men to others,
> sometimes even of one man to all others; and to show also the
> advisability of appointing such person or persons to guide, to lead,
> or on occasion even to compel and subdue, their inferiors according
> to their own better knowledge and wiser will (paragraph 54).

Those who have wondered why, in practice, socialists can be so snobbish
may have their answer here. They were not snobs in spite of being socialists,
in all likelihood, but socialists because they were snobs. Capitalism, after
all, is radically vulgar – 'In trade, my dear . . .' – and it can give spending
power to the most dreadful people. An eminent socialist once remarked in
a supermarket: 'These places make me hate the human race.' The smell of
common humanity repels by doctrine and by instinct; as Ruskin put it, the
aim is to show the eternal superiority of some men to others.

Armies, after all, demonstrate that hierarchy can mean effective order
through collective discipline. In 1931, in his autobiography *My Eighty
Years*, Robert Blatchford, the Victorian journalist, tells how he joined the
army at the age of twenty, in 1871, and 'learned the value of collective
action', only to be shocked at the sight of barefoot children in London
streets and in the black slums of Manchester. Converted by reading a
pamphlet, he realised that socialism was what his army life had encouraged
him to believe in:

> It meant human brotherhood and cooperation. It meant the collective
> action of the Army. It meant *esprit de corps*. . . . (p. 37).

It meant patriotism, too, as military service does. 'The kind of Socialism I
am advocating here is Collectivism', he wrote in 1902, in *Britain for the
British*; since the nation owns the instruments by which it wages war, it
should also own the instruments of production, distribution and property
to make war on inefficiency and destitution. Ruskin's curtsey and hat-
doffing is now a military salute.

The principle of socialist aristocracy was candidly announced by Lenin
fifteen years before he seized power, and in *What Is to Be Done?*, a
pamphlet written in exile, he put a blunt case for the rule of an intellectual
élite. The fate of this highly important work illustrates the incuriosity with
which socialist scriptures are often held, since the most scholarly edition

in English – the Oxford edition of 1963 by S.V. Utechin – is based on a shortened Russian text issued in St Petersburg in 1907, and makes its own further omissions; to consult the full text in English one would have to turn to a version of the Soviet edition of Lenin's works. No doubt Lenin is scarcely more distinguished than Adolf Hitler as a stylist, but his empire was vaster and lasted longer, and the text of *Mein Kampf* has not been treated as cavalierly as this. Lenin's argument is uncompromising. Since Marxist revolution is based on theory, and only intellectuals can understand theory, only an intellectual élite can lead the revolution: 'the educated representatives of the propertied class, the intelligentsia' (II.A). Marx and Engels, after all, as he justly remarks, were bourgeois intellectuals. So, of course, was Lenin; and so, for the most part, were the great Marxist dictators of Europe and Asia after him, like Mao Tse-Tung. Socialism necessarily means government by a privileged class, as Lenin saw, since only those of privileged education are capable of planning and governing. Shaw and Wells, too, often derided the notion that ordinary people can be trusted with political choice. Hence the aristocratic superiority of the Bolsheviks, who reminded Bertrand Russell, when he visited Lenin soon after the October Revolution, of the British public-school élite that then governed India. Socialism had to be based on privilege, and knew it, since only privilege educates for the due exercise of centralised power in a planned economy.

The next step was for the ruling élites of the socialist world to grant themselves the privileges, sometimes even the hereditary privileges, of a ruling caste. Socialism was soon seen to be hereditary in its nature: it conferred unlimited economic power, after all; unlimited economic power means unlimited power, in practice, and rulers who possess that naturally assume personal privileges for themselves and their own. They do not cease to be human because they have made a revolution. The rapidity with which the socialist world formed itself into an *ancien régime* took some observers by surprise, presumably because they had not read Ruskin or Lenin, Shaw or Wells. Stalin's son, who died in a German prisoner-of-war camp, was destined by his father for high office, and knew it; the Rumania of President Ceausescu had his wife and son in the cabinet; Erich Honecker of East Germany gave his wife a cabinet post; and the communist leader of North Korea, Kim Il Sung, founded a dynasty for his relatives. By the 1950s even some communists were admitting that something like the rule of the Bourbons had been restored to much of Europe and large tracts of Asia as well. In 1957 the Yugoslav dissident Milovan Djilas published *The New Class*, a book that shattered the illusions of many – not because it said anything that was new, exactly, but because it was said, and for the first time, by a former member of a communist government. Since socialism gives an administrative monopoly to one party, Djilas argued, the party quickly and inevitably turns into a privileged caste. 'The party makes the class', he wrote, and 'the class grows stronger while the party grows weaker. . . .' The Communist political bureaucracy uses, enjoys and disposes of nationalised property (pp. 40, 44), turning it into a Bourbon-style system of high-living magnates like Tito who pay no taxes and live in palaces, their daily existence eased by chauffeured cars, opera boxes and yachts, not to mention servants and medical care paid for out of the public purse. Socialism readily becomes a system ripe for exploitation by friends and relatives. The example of Sanjay Gandhi, appointed by his mother as head of a state car firm and destined, had he lived, to succeed her as prime minister of India, shows that even in elective systems public ownership and hereditary privilege can go hand in hand.

The majestic conclusion to all this lay in the deification of Lenin and Mao after their deaths, when like ancient emperors or Christian worthies they abandoned the dignity of sages and monarchs to become saints or gods. Lenin was laid in a tomb in Red Square in Moscow, his body-fluids replaced at his death in 1924 by a chemical compound that leaves in doubt whether the object of veneration is Lenin or not, a problem familiar in style to historians of the medieval church.[1] After 1953 Stalin joined him for eight years, an embalmed corpse. When Mao died in 1976 the example was felt to be challenging and, as *China Youth News* revealed in December 1992, more than ten thousand people were involved in designing the sarcophagus, the Communist Party holding a national meeting of coffin-makers where six coffins were judged to be fit for the Great Helmsman of the Chinese people, five of them being kept as spares. The glow on his face, as he lies in a crystal sarcophagus in the Mao museum in Peking, is now known to have been achieved by running light-conducting fibres into the sarcophagus, so that the light is reflected on his features, carefully arranged to disguise his wrinkles. This leaves all other instances of saint-worship since the early Christians looking jejune and paltry.

It will be asked why, if socialists could declare themselves to be Tory, they were not condemned by radical and liberal opinion.

The answer is that they were, though the debate is now forgotten. Shortly after Marx and Engels issued *The Communist Manifesto* in 1848 a youthful Adolphe Thiers, one day to be President of the French Republic, wrote a pamphlet called *Du Communisme*, where he concluded that any attempt to abolish private property would destroy incentives to work and create still more poverty; by frustrating the hopes of the poor, he argued, socialism would in the end kill liberty and strengthen tyranny. At the same time a radical lawyer, Alfred Sudre, issued a remarkable book now wholly unread, though it went

---

1. See Nina Tumarkin, *Lenin Lives: the Lenin Cult in Soviet Russia*

through several editions in its day and was crowned with a prize by the French Academy. Sudre does not even mention Marx or Engels in his *Histoire du Communisme*, but he traces the history of the idea from Plato through Sir Thomas More to Proudhon, concluding that since Plato's time socialism had always been 'an obstacle to progress' by replacing liberty with the rule of despots. Five years later, in a sequel on sovereignty, he condemned ancient Greek influence on the modern mind for its fatal dedication to *a priori* reasoning – what Sudre called 'its fierce determination to realise, at whatever cost, the conceptions of arrogant theorising'. These are liberal protests, in the wake of the revolution of 1848, against the predictably conservative effects of socialist theories. In a later chapter I shall attempt to place these arguments in the context of revolutionary events in Paris in 1848.

Sudre's conclusion in 1849, in his history of communism, was passionate and eloquent. He had been active for the parliamentary cause in the recent revolution, he explains, with the overthrow of the July monarchy in February 1848, and had written his book as a warning against the socialist agitation that the violent creation of the Second French Republic had just witnessed. Almost nothing, unfortunately, is known about him. A Parisian lawyer, he is said to have been born in 1820, so that he was still in his twenties when he wrote his first book and won his Academy prize; and he argued that attacks on private property have always been reactionary in effect and commonly so in purpose. Ancient Sparta, for example, which (unlike Athens) divided the land into equal portions and proscribed monied property, left its citizens in brute ignorance and trained them only for wars that devastated and enslaved their neighbours. Socialism, he wrote, has always been

> an obstacle to progress, has slowed its pace and harnessed itself
> backwards to the chariot of civilisation. Humanity has advanced
> not because of socialism but in spite of it, developing rather by the
> gradual extension of property and liberty, of equality of rights and
> legal enactments, by the progressive enhancement and purification
> of the principles of marriage and the family; by science, literature
> and the arts.

Communism necessarily means regression. It has

> tried to suppress all those elements of progress and in their place
> set despotism, equality of degradation, promiscuity and ignorance.
> All the great revolutions have been achieved outside communism:
> the abolition of slavery, the liberation of the human spirit that man-
> kind owes to the Reformation, to Galileo, Bacon and Descartes; the
> abolition of feudalism and of inequalities before the law achieved
> on the night of 4th August (pp. 478-9)

when titles and feudal rights were abolished by the French National

Assembly in 1789. Sudre was passionately certain that socialism was a reactionary idea. It is a pity that no known document reveals precisely which political parties or groups he knew or watched in the tumultuous events in Paris in 1848; but his book, still unknown in English but translated into German in 1882 in an extended form, was once famous or at least known, and Lord Acton owned two copies of it in different editions. Since his death, which may have occurred in the mid 1880s, he has unfortunately suffered the oblivion that sometimes befalls minds of inconvenient perceptions and embarrassing convictions.

It is sometimes thought, for all that, that socialism in its day at least bequeathed to Europe and elsewhere the blessings of the welfare state.

That is not how it appeared at the time. The welfare enactments of the Liberal government of 1906-14, promoted by Asquith, Lloyd George and Churchill, were an outcome not of socialism but of a New Liberalism to which the small parliamentary group of Labour members, intent only on trade-union reform, had to be persuaded.[1] Nor did William Beveridge, the author of National Health Service in Britain, think kindly of socialism, and often complained in his last years of the resistance of Labour leaders during the second world war to his Report of 1942. 'I joined the Liberal Party', he once told a public meeting, 'and sat in the Commons as a Liberal, for two reasons: one, that I was and am a Liberal; and two, that the Liberals were the only party that wholeheartedly welcomed my plans for a National Health Service'. In his memoir *Power and Influence* he left a record of Ernest Bevin's opposition as a Labour leader:

> For Ernest Bevin, with his trade-union background of unskilled workers, . . . social insurance was less important than bargaining about wages (p. 295),

recalling how Bevin had derided the Beveridge Report as a 'Social Ambulance Scheme', and how furious he had been when back-bench Labour members ignored their leaders and voted for it in February 1943. That capitalism, once rendered humane, might also be rendered harmless, even popular, was a profound and intelligible fear of the socialist mind in the early years of the century. Events have proved it right. When the two Germanies were united in 1990-1, the welfare provision of the capitalist West was discovered to be more than twice that of the socialist East, and it was the realisation that it takes a free market to sustain public welfare through massive wealth-creation that powerfully contributed to the death of socialism in the last years of the twentieth century.

---

1. See Peter Clarke, *Liberals and Social Democrats*

5
Tocqueville's Burden of Liberty

A novel can seize on the spirit of the age; and such a novel was Trollope's *The Warden* of 1855, with which he achieved his first success at forty.

The Warden tells the story of a scrupulously honourable old clergyman, the Reverend Septimus Harding of Barchester, who innocently accepts a sinecure at the hands of his ecclesiastical superiors – the comfortable wardenship of an old men's home – till he is rudely forced by a press campaign to give it up. "The tenth Muse", as Trollope contemptuously called journalism, thunders like Jupiter from Mount Olympus and hounds the kindly old cleric into a resignation from which everyone suffers, even the pensioners. The plot is a paradigm of moderate Victorian thought in the middle decades of the century and of a good deal of debate since, for it concerns the burden of liberty, a doctrine whose ultimate source is likely to be Tocqueville's *Democracy in America* (1835-40); and the exquisite tragedy that lies at the heart of the first Barchester novel lies in Trollope's acknowledgement that, while everyone has suffered from Mr Harding's resignation, an act of intense moral perfection has yet been performed. The novel celebrates what Iris Murdoch has called 'the for-nothingness of good'. It is very anti-Utilitarian. Good acts can diminish human happiness on all sides and yet remain good.

The theme of a joyless and envy-ridden liberty was recurrent in the fiction of the age in which socialism was born. Dickens attempted something like it six years after Trollope, in *Great Expectations*, a novel about a self-promoting youth called Pip eager to be a gentleman who wins what he wants only at bitter cost to his tranquillity and self-respect. George Eliot was already applying the principle to the still more acute case of womankind. In her last two novels, especially – in *Middlemarch* and *Daniel Deronda* – self-willed young women make bad choices in marriage and are punished for it: punished, so to speak, by their freedom. The principle is a major element in Turgenev's fiction; and Ibsen was to embody it in three dramatic masterpieces – *The Wild Duck, Rosmersholm* and *Hedda Gabler* – where a liberty to know the truth, the dangerous whole truth, destroys those who innocently imagine that sexual emancipation can only be a blessing. By the 1890s Henry James, in *What Maisie Knew* and *The Turn of the Screw*, extends the principle to the young, even the childish – he turns the screw, as he puts it, to make it a child that sees a truth it cannot bear, and gives it 'two turns' by adding a second child; and the reader is meant to guess, through a thin veil of dark hints, that (like Ibsen's

Hedda) James's two children have learned the facts of life too soon, so that in the last paragraph little Miles appears to die of knowledge, so to speak, in the arms of his governess.

It is less this body of fiction itself I want to consider here than its analytical sources. It represents an impressively dark side of Victorian liberalism – a side neglected, even denied, by many modern critics, who have often preferred to see the age as glibly and naively optimistic. My theme here is the tragic dimension of the liberal idea, and of the first great analyst of that new dimension, Alexis de Tocqueville, who wrote when socialism was barely a word.

All these authors were liberals. They were in no sense attacking freedom of commerce or of thought, in the end, merely lifting a warning finger against its foreseeable human perils. It is the tragic strength of their position that they never abandon faith; their critique is always conducted from inside a system of belief, never against it. They warn rather than demolish. The rascally and uncaring radical journalists who overturn the prosperity and peace of mind of good men and women in Trollope's novels or Ibsen's plays are, after all, abusing a freedom which in law is justly theirs: the right to print. Dorothea Brooke's high-minded knowledge of the world of scholarship, in *Middlemarch*, oddly precocious and gravely damaging as it proves, or Hedda Gabler's prurient fascination with Løvborg's seedy nightlife, are a natural outcome of free publishing and free conversation. Young ladies, even children, get to know things. James was to embody the problem in its conversational aspects in another Nineties novel tellingly entitled *The Awkward Age*, which concerns the delicate problem of girls too old to be treated as children but still too young to be freely bantered with. Liberalism removed a straitjacket from the advanced social life of western Europe and North America in the middle decades of the nineteenth century; and its ideals of free trade and free thought were inextricably mingled, as the age knew, if only because books and newspapers arecommodities to be bought and sold. But freedom leaves people free to make mistakes, whether in business, friendship or love; and those mistakes, like Pip's or Dorothea's, are now bluntly their own fault. So the liberal world does not easily allow for self-excusing, as socialism would one day do and as the hierarchical old world had done. Freedom spells responsibility, responsibility error, and error the oppressive guilt of error.

Yet there is no going back; and the burden of liberty would be worth no analysis at all if the new world could return to an old one where thought was unfree, stations in life fixed, and young women bound to accept parental advice about whom to marry. It is a firm assumption of these novels, plays and treatises that we cannot return; and liberalism, unlike socialism, is not nostalgic. Liberal man, like Milton's fallen Adam, is now free to wander, anywhere except where he came from. That is why his new freedom, imperative as it is, is a source of anxiety. He can get it wrong, as never before; and yet he can neither lose the memory of an ordered paradise of hierarchy and obedience nor hope to recover it.

Tocqueville's *Democracy in America* appeared in 1835-40, to instant and enormous acclaim in France and England. It was a report by a young French aristocrat who had travelled on official business in the United States in 1831-2, and it brought its author fame, honour and membership of the French Academy. Lord Acton was to call him 'always wise, always right, and as just as Aristides'; and a century later Denis Brogan called *Democracy in America* the best book ever written about the United States and its political system. But it has seldom been read through, except by specialists, perhaps because its fastidiously aristocratic liberalism has appealed little to twentieth-century tastes. As early as *Fabian Essays*, published in 1889, Sidney Webb called the book 'a classic which everyone quotes and nobody reads'. We have lately preferred dark, superstitious cult-theories concerning the sociology of thought emanating from forests east of the Rhine; and even the French, until recently, have preferred the dense jungles of Marx and his successors to the more lucid light cast on them from nearer home, though a biography of Tocqueville by André Jardin was the talk of literary Paris in 1984. But as the Marxian cult ends, the long task of reclaiming the intelligentsia of the West for liberty has begun, and Tocqueville is among its inspirations. The omens are set fair. His civilised clarity of mind suddenly looks engagingly new to a generation brought up on the brouhaha of May 1968 and its long aftermath of disillusion. Political violence daily loses its romance through the sheer familiarity of terror; strikes have made too many headlines in the industrial West to allow the myth of class war to look anything better, by now, than antiquated and quaint; and where class hatreds have failed of achievement, rationality may prevail. 'Wise, right, and just', Acton called Tocqueville; and the spectacle of a lover of liberty who may have been all three takes on a sudden, wilful charm.

And some surprises. Most surprising of all is Tocqueville's dark view that individual liberty might in the end prove problematical and burdensome. It was a view that took instant hold both in England and in America. *Democracy in America* was translated into English as soon as it appeared, and was promptly and avidly read on both sides of the Atlantic; on his second visit to England in 1835 Tocqueville was eagerly fêted there, meeting John Stuart Mill and beginning a long correspondence with him. George Henry Lewes, the future companion of George Eliot, met him in Paris in 1842, armed with an introduction from Mill himself. Gladstone tells in his diary (8 August 1849) how he dined with him there seven years later, at the British Embassy, when Tocqueville was briefly the Foreign Secretary of France. In old age, according to John Morley, Gladstone described Tocqueville as 'the nearest French approach to Burke'. By then Tocqueville had been dead for over thirty years. But he had generously called England 'intellectually my second country'; and as he lay dying in the south of France in 1859 a copy of Mill's essay *On Liberty* reached him, sent on by its admiring author. Too weak to read it, in all likelihood, he may yet have felt that a torch had been passed.

Tocqueville had taught Mill, among others, to see liberty as a dangerous responsibility to be borne rather than a right to be claimed and enjoyed. He was the author of mature liberalism, so to speak, as opposed to the utopian liberalism of Shelley and Byron, which was to have no future in the parliamentary state that followed their death by a few years with the first Reform Act of 1832. In his *Autobiography* of 1873 Mill acknowledged Tocqueville as the man who had shifted him from a naive belief in 'pure democracy' to that 'modified form of it' he had cautiously expounded in *Representative Government*. Modified democratic sentiment is based on sober fear of what Mill, echoing Tocqueville, calls the 'tyranny of the majority', along with a dread of centralisation based on what Tocqueville had seen of its effects in France. Tocqueville's fear of centralisation was soon to be Mill's and Gladstone's, and it is a fundamentally anti-socialist view. Unless the powers of government can be curbed, the drive towards equality of condition could lead to the worst tyranny there could ever be: 'the absolute rule of the head of the executive', as Mill put it in the *Autobiography*, 'over a congregation of isolated individuals, all equals but all slaves'. When Napoleon III took power in France in November 1852 as emperor, less than a year after his democratic election as a republican president in December 1851, it must have seemed to Tocqueville a grim, belated illustration of his point, and for the last seven years of his life he lived in retirement from French public life and even from France, composing the *Ancien Régime* and exchanging letters with like-minded men in England and at home.

As early as 1835, when he reviewed *Democracy in America*, Mill had seen the point of Tocqueville's predictions about the forward march of the new world. The task now, as he remarked in his review, was less to welcome it than to prepare: 'not to determine whether democracy shall come, but how to make the best of it when it does come, is the scope of M. de Tocqueville's speculations.' On his return from America, Tocqueville had offered the world an alarming vision of a place where, as he put it, 'the spell of royalty is broken, but has not been succeeded by the majesty of the laws', and where a shift towards equality of condition in the non-slave states was intensifying individual hatreds. All that represents a polar opposite to utopian liberalism:

> The division of property has lessened the distance which separated
> the rich from the poor; but . . . the nearer they draw to each other,
> the greater is their mutual hatred, and the more vehement the envy
> and the dread with which they resist each other's claims to power.

Civil liberty, he feared, could all too easily turn joyless. Whereas in unreformed Europe he saw placid faces and light spirits, Americans in the 1830s had 'a cloud habitually hung upon their brow' and took their pleasures sadly, 'forever brooding over advantages they do not possess'.

The point is arresting in itself and characteristic of its century. History had dealt two new cards into the pack – democracy and industrialism – and by the 1830s both were imminent, if not actually present. Democracy here means male adult suffrage moving – as many believed it must – towards ever greater equality of condition; and it was that alarming tendency that was the main theme of Tocqueville's great book. 'America was only the frame, democracy the picture', as he put it. In the American states without slavery he had seen the future, and it worked – but not as one might wish. Democracy was wormed in the bud.

Industrialism, however, that other new card and the chief impulse of the socialist idea, he treats of hardly at all, as if outside his brief. By the 1830s only Britain was an industrial state, though some of its techniques were beginning to pass to the Continent and North America. By hindsight, at least, industry now looks as vast in its after-effects as democracy, since it made of poverty, in the strict sense – starvation and homelessness – a choice and an option for the first time. The first growing-pains past, peaceful industrial nations in favourable circumstances can reasonably hope to abolish starvation and homelessness, if they choose; and individuals, if they choose, can reasonably hope to be prosperous and educated. That is the choice that Dickens's Pip and George Eliot's Dorothea Brooke make as individuals, in *Great Expectations* and *Middlemarch*: it is not one imposed on them by family or by nature, as it would have been in a novel by Fielding or Jane Austen. No age of mankind had contemplated anything like it before those decisive decades that elapsed between Waterloo and the revolutions of 1848. Men can choose: the thought was enough to make a radical out of anyone. It was in those thirty years and more that the modern political choice of conservative, socialist and liberal was born.

The choice needs pondering. Before the Enlightenment popular liberty had been too remote a prospect to excite much in the way of fear or hope; and since the first world war the fear of liberty has become something like a taboo. Jean-Paul Sartre tried to revive it in the guise of existentialist agony in the 1940s: but modern political systems have usually rejected it,

at least in name and in rhetoric. Even dictatorships have often taken care
to describe themselves as democracies, or People's Democracies; and ifany-
one is afraid of freedom nowadays it is highly unusual to hear him say so.

Tocqueville's shrewd point confers a uniqueness on *Democracy in
America*, then, and on the controversy it immediately provoked: the more
so because, like his friend Mill, he was to live and die a lover of liberty.
Their critique of democracy was never meant as a dismissal. It was meant,
rather, to engage attentions more critically, as men might brace themselves
for a crisis they will soon have to face. All that was radically different
from the mood of the first French revolutionaries after 1789, who failed
because they had been unwilling to count the cost of liberty to human
happiness until it had been paid – and radically unlike the fervent libertarian
mood of the young Wordsworth or the young Shelley. The 1830sinaugurated
a new phase in the march of the liberal idea: more searching, more empirical
in its use of evidence since (unlike its predecessors) it now had practical
evidence of popular liberty to use; and above all cautiously, even pessi-
mistically, anti-utopian. A parliamentary idea, in fact, rather than an idea
for revolutionary cliques or assemblies: one thing at a time.

It was a sense of caution that suited the France of the July monarchy
after 1830 and the England of the first Reform Bill, introduced into the
Commons in the same year. Tocqueville's book came in due season. 'In
much wisdom is much grief', said Ecclesiastes, 'and he that increaseth
knowledge increaseth sorrow'. That might remind one of the wail of Henry
James's governess for the children in her charge in *The Turn of the Screw*:
'They know, they know!' The new mood of Tocqueville and Mill was not
quite as dark as that; but neither did it hold out easy hopes of a human
nature newly born again. Men are irreversibly what they are, regardless of
laws and constitutions, and what they are they will remain: greedy, envious
and fallible. Any theory that neglects that is a cloudy fantasy, and it is for
the political theorist to learn at last to cut his cloth to man as he is.

But what is he? He is, at all events, a creature that needs to be guided and
ruled, however constitutionally free within the limits of law. He can be
oppressed by freedom. 'Thank goodness we don't have to *choose*
tomorrow', I once overheard one schoolchild remark to another on the
way home one afternoon, presumably from a progressive school. A modern
housewife is blessed by consumer choice, on the whole; but in the biggest
supermarkets her choices can be baffling and even agonising. The super-
market puts the burden of liberty at its easiest. At its hardest, an openly
competitive system can crush the individual, as Mill and Tocqueville first
saw, with a sense of purely personal failure: he no longer has the excuse
once afforded by an *ancien régime* of being called by God or King to an

unchanging status in life, from cradle to grave. Modern feminism has claimed to have achieved something of similar effect, in recent years, for some women: with open access to higher education for both sexes, for example, women can no longer readily hold the system itself to blame if they fail to reach good degrees or good jobs; and with no system to blame, they blame themselves.

That disturbing conclusion was clearly seen by Tocqueville's first English translator, Henry Reeve. A future editor of the *Edinburgh Review*, he was a man far less intelligent than Mill. But when he issued a translation of the first volume of *Democracy in America* in the year of its appearance, in 1835, he clearly saw that it was epoch-making, and why. The age of Machiavelli's *Prince*, he announced in his preface, was ending; its sequel being not yet ready.

> The book of "The Prince" is closed forever as a state manual; and
> the book of "The People" is as yet unwritten,

as he put it portentously. Autocracy is dead or dying, that is, and democracy, though probably inescapable, has not yet arrived. But when it does, Reeve warns, it may be no less grim than Machiavelli's famous book: 'of perhaps darker sophistries and more pressing tyranny'. Liberty will exact its human price.

The warning was one Mill sought to enlarge throughout his life as a political theorist. The progress of mankind, as he saw it, depended on diversity, even eccentricity; and democracy threatened that diversity if it brought equality with it. China, he argues in his essay *On Liberty*, though blessed with a high civilisation, has remained 'stationary' for thousands of years, whereas Europe has so far saved itself from a Chinese uniformity by its 'diversity of character and culture' and by the plurality of paths it has followed. But now the writing is on the wall, and it is democracy that is inscribing it there:

> M. de Tocqueville, in his last important work, remarks how much
> more the Frenchmen of the present day resemble one another than
> did those even of the last generation. The same remark might be
> made of Englishmen in a far greater degree,

for though there is greater freedom there is also, by an assimilation of social ranks, a diminishing 'variety of situations'. Written a century before television became commonplace, Mill's charge against the habits of ordinary citizens and their innate tendency to homogenise needs by now to be redoubled:

> Comparatively speaking, they now read the same things, listen to
> the same things, see the same things, go to the same places, have
> their hopes and fears directed to the same objects;

and he adds, in horror of the imminent prospect of the approaching equality of mass-production and democracy, that 'the assimilation is still proceeding', since political changes have recently tended 'to raise the low and to lower the high', notably through free trade and wider education. The coming danger to liberty is equality – equality of condition.

Mill's horror of equality is Gladstonian. He was to sit in the Commons as a Gladstonian Member of Parliament from 1865 to 1868, when his leader finally became Prime Minister, voting obediently on the liberal side; and Gladstone's horror of equality was a byword in his age, though the argument has since dropped from view. That makes of Gladstonism, by now, a highly instructive curiosity. No political party or group in our times openly demands inequality of condition; so that this aspect of Victorian liberalism, largely forgotten as it now is, might be called mind-enlarging. It is an active principle in the fiction of Dickens, Thackeray and George Eliot, who openly celebrate social differences and disparage mechanical nostrums like the suffrage – George Eliot's *Felix Holt* of 1866 is the classic instance – as if they felt social uniformity to be as great a threat to human progress as aristocracy or monarchy had once been. The danger is that if you give the masses freedom to choose, they may all want the same thing. The whole world could turn into California.

The crucial English debate for and against equality began shortly before 1879, when Gladstone won the Midlothian by-election for the Liberals and returned in triumph to the Commons; and it ended in 1889 with the *Fabian Essays* of Bernard Shaw and others. The liberal leader had thrown down a defiant challenge to socialism. He was openly opposed to equality of condition and proudly called himself an Inequalitarian – a word which, no doubt rightly, he believed he had invented.[1] Mill, meanwhile, on his death in 1873, had left certain "Chapters on Socialism", to be published posthumously in the *Fortnightly Review* in the very year of Gladstone's return to Parliament; and a year before, Matthew Arnold had contributed an article on "Equality" to the same journal. The fight was on, and not only ideologically. Reprinted in his *Mixed Essays*, Arnold's essay derisively quoted Gladstone, whom he hated, to the effect that 'equality was utterly unattractive to the people of this country' and inequality 'so dear to their hearts' that egalitarianism was always happily foredoomed to fail. In all that Gladstone was a Millite. Communism, Mill had written years before in his *Principles of Political Economy* of 1848, can never leave any asylum for 'individuality of character'; so that an unpropertied society could only prove 'a tyrannical yoke'.[2] That communism must prove tyrannical, by its nature, was clear to the greatest British liberal theorist as early as 1848,

---

1. W.E. Gladstone, *Gleanings* vol. 1 p. 234
2. Mill revised this section (II.i.3) intensively, though without radical change of argument. See his *Principles*, edited by J.M. Robson, p. 1xxiv

the year of revolutions and of Marx's *Communist Manifesto*. It cannot sensibly be argued, then, that liberal theory was taken unawares by the socialist case in the 1840s, or that it allowed it to pass unanswered. By its very nature, it believed, the search for equality is despotic and unprogressive.

Mill's answer, like Tocqueville's before him, was a salutary warning to the West; and the West, it may be nervously suggested, has appeared to heed it. Social equality is not now an active hope or fear in America or in western Europe – and still less, paradoxically, in China or what was once the Soviet Union. The reasons are hard to pinpoint, and it would be rash to fix them on a single argument. Scepticism about high taxes in the cause of undiscriminating welfare has mounted; millions imagine, and perhaps rightly, that an equal share of little is less exciting, as a prospect, than a larger share of more. Life is a lottery, and should be. For whatever reason, the West has not gone what Mill once called Chinese, or what a recent song has called Ticky-Tacky. In spite of democracy and advancing industrialism, we remain – most of us – individually distinct: we look different, and seek no less ardently to distinguish ourselves; and what Rousseau once memorably called 'la fureur de se distinguer' grows no less. Whether mankind has been helped, in all that, by Tocqueville's warning a century and a half ago is unclear. But certainly the voice of that great Frenchman, 'wise, right and just', who in the end saw as much to hope for as to fear in the democratic experiment, no longer sounds lonely or unheard in America or in his native land.

6

The Forgotten French of 1848

'A spectre is haunting Europe', wrote Karl Marx in *The Communist Manifesto* of 1848, in one of the most famous opening sentences of political literature, and the spectre was communism.

The pamphlet, exceptionally happy in its timing, was written in Brussels in the first weeks of 1848, the year of revolutions, by an obscure Rhineland insurrectionary not yet thirty. It was promptly published in the original German in London in February, in a highly inaccurate edition of about a thousand copies, to be corrected, translated and reprinted for a century and more; and it deserved its success, since it summarises with pungency and uncharacteristic brevity views that Marx and Engels – who helped Marx with advice – had already made public. Its fame rests less on its novelty, then, than on its style. It set the tone, in literary terms, for the year of revolutions, and no socialist tract (it seems reasonable to guess) has been more widely read. Europe was about to explode.

France was the European nation most radically affected by the violence of 1848. On 24th February the July monarchy of Louis-Philippe was violently overthrown, ushering in the short and troubled life of the Second Republic. A few weeks later, in March, Metternich fell from power in Vienna, though the Austrian imperial system survived his fall. History was being made at high speed, and Marx's bold talk about the spectre of communism was not bravado. Even before 1848 Europe, and above all France, already had reason to fear the violence of worker-revolution.

It was in the mid-1830s that the atmosphere had changed. George Sand remarked in *Horace*, her novel of 1842, that in the early 1830s 'people were not afraid, as they are today, to be thought communist', whereas now the word had become 'a bogey to all shades of opinion'. Secret republican clubs were active in Paris by the mid-1830s; in 1839 Blanqui attempted an armed revolt, which was easily suppressed; while advanced republicans like Cavaignac were demanding universal suffrage, free education and a redistribution of property. It was in Paris, where the young Marx arrived in November 1843, that he became a communist, and there, only months later, that he met Engels. Socialism and communism, its more violent rival, may not have been French inventions, but it was in France that they first took root. The terms, it seems likely, were English, so that it was the English who conceived, the Germans who theorised and the French who took to the streets. Socialism was first used as a term by Robert Owen in the *Cooperative Magazine* in 1827; and it was an English Christian Socialist, Goodwyn Barmby, who claimed in 1848 to have invented the word 'communism' in Paris in 1840. But what Owen and Barmby did belongs to lexicography rather than to political history, and there is no doubt that by the 1840s both dogmas looked French. No other large nation, as early as that, harboured violent groups devoted to social revolution and capable, as February 1848 showed, of changing governments and constitutions by demonstrations and riots, and it was a riot outside and inside the Chamber of Deputies in that month that finally toppled the monarchy. Shortly afterwards the new republic introduced male adult suffrage, the first on earth, and debated, though usually without adopting, statutes that threatened the rights of property. In July Proudhon's proposal to suspend and reduce all rents was rejected. The atmosphere in the summer of 1848 was heady with the prospect of social change, and it was in those dangerous months that two Frenchmen, Adolphe Thiers and Alfred Sudre, wrote their treatises in defence of private ownership.

What they wrote, unlike *The Communist Manifesto*, is now forgotten, but they deserve as thinkers to be remembered. By 1848 Thiers was a fifty-year-old man of some property, and had twice been prime minister under the monarchy. During the summer he wrote a series of articles for the *Constitutionnel* which he collected as *De la Propriété*, the preface being dated September 1848; he apologises there for having taken so long to write the book among the distractions of a political life and his work as an historian. However, he adds, the argument had been revolving in his head for some years, and he marshals it analytically: first a defence of the right to private property, followed by chapters attacking first socialism and then communism. One day to become the first president of the Third Republic, Thiers was already a famous man, and the book was promptly translated into English as *The Rights of Property: a Refutation of Communism and Socialism*, with extensive historical notes added by an unknown translator.

Some weeks later a young Paris lawyer called Alfred Sudre published a *Histoire du Communisme*, its preface dated 1st November. This was the first history of socialism (or communism) in any language, and it was written, as the preface explains, during the confused events of the summer of 1848 and, to all appearances, without reference to Thiers's book or to *The Communist Manifesto*, which was not yet available in French. Sudre was born two years after Marx, in 1820, but unlike Marx he remains an obscure figure. In the preface of his first book he speaks of being called to arms, presumably as a member of the National Guard in the streets of Paris in June 1848 in defence of the social verities (as he calls them) that his history is concerned to justify; and the book is erudite in its handling of ancient sources, though he may have had little leisure to read the pamphlets of the day. It is natural to assume that *The Communist Manifesto* and the works of Thiers and Sudre derive not from one another, then, but from a common body of arguments for and against private property in the France of the 1840s. Only the German pamphlet, however, is now remembered. France was the cradle of socialism in the 1840s under the July monarchy, and of its more violent extreme known as communism. But in literary terms the French of 1848 are now forgotten.

The fall of the monarchy in February, as Sudre explains, was a surprise. Much as Guizot, Louis-Philippe's conservative prime minister, was detested, the constitution itself was not widely expected to fall, and within days of its fall it was clear that a fate even more perilous than universal male suffrage threatened France – a threat to property itself. Socialism and communism, Sudre argues, had gained an influence in the 1840s rashly ignored by enlightened opinion, and his book, which must have been written in a rush, though perhaps from historical materials already assembled, was a belated attempt to answer the arguments of communism that had once seemed too rash and too silly to need answering at all. It is a pioneering attempt to trace a subversive body of theories back to their sources in the fatal utopianism of the ancient Greeks, as theorised in Plato's *Republic* and practised in Sparta. In ancient Sparta the land was equally divided by area among its free citizens and worked by helots or slaves. Plato, meanwhile, proposed a utopia ruled by a just élite to whom property and marriage are forbidden: the first blueprint, as Sudre sees it, of more recent and still more dangerous attempts to define and institute a perfect state. His story continues through the early Christians, the German Anabaptists of the sixteenth century, and Sir Thomas More's *Utopia* of 1516. Then it turns mainly French, with chapters on the eighteenth-century philosophers, the French Revolution of 1789 and the egalitarian doctrines of Babeuf, who was guillotined in 1797; and it ends with accounts of early nineteenth-century theorists such as Robert Owen, Saint-Simon and Charles Fourier, along with Louis Blanc and Proudhon. The book takes no interest in Germany since the Reformation, and though it appeared some nine months or more after *The Communist Manifesto* it does not mention Engels or Marx. That had to wait till a German version in 1882, when the book was extensively expanded by Otto Wenzel.

An historical plan must seem remarkable for a doctrine which as early as the 1840s had no very continuous ancestry, but the book is less an academic treatise than a polemic in the shape of a history. That is announced on the title-page, with the subtitle "an historical refutation of socialist utopias". Sudre accepts the challenge of historical interpretation and the analysis of ancient and medieval sources. Even before he wrote the *Histoire*, socialists and communists were already given to justifying their views by appeals to the Ancients as well as to primitive Christians and medieval heretics; years later, in fact, Engels was to remark disapprovingly that French socialists were nearly all Christians, and in his *Catéchisme des Socialistes* of 1849 Louis Blanc bluntly called socialism 'the gospel in action'. Socialism was always, in one way or another, a theory of history, and it is historical parallels like these that Sudre debates, unaware that Marx and Engels had already linked the coming revolution to a bold and comprehensive theory of class war.

His arguments, none the less, can be placed in a French context, if the pamphlets of the age are examined. An undated pamphlet by the Catholic apologist Frédéric Ozanam, for example, *Les Origines du Socialisme*, may already have appeared. Ozanam died in 1853, and two years later the pamphlet was collected in the seventh volume of his *Oeuvres*. True, its religious element marks it out, as an anti-socialist argument, from Sudre's entirely secular view. But some of his points prefigure Sudre's, notably his claim that socialism represents not progress but a return to the past. Socialist doctrines, he argues, have never been nearer fulfilment than in the theocratic nations of antiquity, like ancient India or Persia, or in Plato's *Republic*, which had implied the abolition of private property. Ozanam's pamphlet traverses much of the same ground as Sudre's book: Sudre's thesis too is that the abolition or equalisation of private property, as in Platonic theory or Spartan practice, must favour the powerful and the rich. The notion that socialism must prove conservative in its effects perhaps starts here, in this forgotten Parisian debate, and it is disarming to see a view Arthur Koestler and George Orwell discovered for themselves in the 1940s laid down so uncompromisingly by obscure Frenchmen a century before. Perhaps the essential conservatism of the socialist idea is a truth that every generation has to discover for itself.

Sudre, in any case, was less an original thinker than the spokesman of a party hitherto content to leave its views unpublished. Like Thiers he held that private property, far from oppressing the poor, was their best defence against oppression, much like Naboth's vineyard in the Book of Kings. Property protects the poor. The powerful scarcely need to own anything, after all, since (like high party officials in the heyday of the Soviet Union) they command the use of what the state provides. The liberating claims of socialism, then, however sincere, are a chimera, and the nation that places economic power in the hands of a central authority, Sudre argues, will end with a tyranny like Plato's guardians, ruled by fear under military discipline. Though the guardians own nothing, they dispose of everything. Such, Sudre argues, was Plato's legacy in his search for perfection. It was the commitment of political thinkers in antiquity to the concept of a perfect state that led them into the monstrous errors that now threaten mankind, and Sudre may have been the first to notice how deeply indebted the early socialist thinkers were to the heritage of ancient philosophy, though his target was not Aristotle, who inspired Marx, but Aristotle's master Plato. It was the search for utopia, Sudre insists, that led Plato to propose the abolition of the family along with communism in property, free abortion and infanticide: all due to the fatal Greek fascination with *a priori* reasoning, or the illusion that the manners and customs of a whole people can be transformed and perfected by laws, that tradition and historical precedent count for nothing.

Sudre's own positive convictions, which remain obscure, were more radical than traditionalist. He was not, apparently, a conservative. Indeed he was anti-socialist because he believed socialism to be conservative. But he is clear that societies have their own momentum and that history has its power to teach. His case is both theoretical and practical. The real charge against communism is that, whatever its motives, its effects would be to create a privileged caste. It is more conservative, as an idea, than any group or party which, in a democratic age, chooses to call itself that.

Such arguments look interesting, but there is not much evidence that they did so at the time. The book went through several editions, it is true, but its critical effects are hard to trace. Though awarded the Prix Montyon by the French Academy when it first appeared, and translated twice into Spanish and, much later, into German, it is not known to have attracted many reviews and was never translated into English. Proudhon in his notebooks exclaimed indignantly about the scale of the prize, which was three thousand francs, and all for a book full of outworn platitudes, as he puts it: 'les mêmes platitudes ressassées'. Perhaps he meant he had already encountered some of Sudre's arguments in the *Constitutionnel*. But his comment, brief and dismissive as it is, stands alone. No historian of socialism, even in France, has ever bothered with the book, in its own century or since, though Elie Halévy, who lectured on European socialism in Paris shortly before his death in 1937, would surely have found it significant. His *Histoire du Socialisme Européen*, published years later in 1948 from notes taken down by his pupils, fails to mention it. Sudre's book sank without a trace; and though Lord Acton owned two copies and marked them, he never mentions it in his writings.

Even Sudre's later career, apart from books on sovereignty and banking, is mysterious. So are his political affiliations, though he may be presumed to have been hostile to the Second Empire instituted by Louis Napoleon in 1852, resigning from the Paris bar on 26th December; and he ends his *Histoire de la Souveraineté* with a long diatribe against the imperial idea in antiquity, condemning an age that can prefer Sparta to Athens and deploring the reign of the Caesars in ancient Rome. The shift from republic to empire, Sudre argues in his final chapter, after an extensive summary of Hebrew, Greek and Roman views of sovereignty, was a shift to decadence, whether in political and military terms or in literary achievement, and Rome here is no doubt a metaphor for France:

> What an enormous difference between what the republic and the empire achieved in the field of politics! The first had conquered the world in a long series of victories, the second could barely keep what had been conquered, and ultimately succumbed less from the effects of the barbarians than from its own weakness. Once caesarism had taken hold, there was no more a senate firm and far-seeing, there were no more great generals or negotiators.

No more great eloquence, either, among the Romans, as in the days of Cicero; indeed human dignity itself, Sudre argues, was degraded by the cult of the imperial title. An age accustomed to parallels between the ancient and the modern would no doubt have read this as a coded rejection of the rule of the Emperor Napoleon III. It seems probable, then, that Sudre, like Thiers, and perhaps with a similar reluctance, accepted the claims of the Second Republic to represent the people of France and regretted its collapse in 1852. He may even have been something of an ideological republican, as Thiers was not, a principled enthusiast for a land without kings and emperors, though surely with something less than the republican zeal of Proudhon or George Sand. Enthusiasm, in any case, was not the mark of his mind, which was lawyer-like and analytical. But he remains an unknown being outside his writings. Even his death, which may have been around 1885, is unrecorded, and his last work – dated March 1882 – appears to have been an affectionate tribute to his dead brother Charles.[1]

Thiers, by contrast, was a famous man by 1848, and in his writings of that year he showed himself little interested in the history or prehistory of the socialist idea. His *Rights of Property* was an analysis of the challenge to property provoked by the French Revolution of 1789, of which in the 1820s, under the Restoration, he had already written an ample history: and though a professional historian, unlike Sudre, all his essays in defence of property are concerned with his own age. France, after all, was the only nation with universal male suffrage and with a recent tradition of violent popular revolution, and nowhere but in France did radical mobs take to the streets and overthrow established dynasties. In Spain the people were conservative, in England peaceful, and in 1848 Germany and Italy were

---

1. Charles Sudre, *Les Finances de la France au XIXe Siècle*, with a preface by Alfred that condemns Napoleon III and praises Gladstone

not yet nations. As the English translator of the book remarks, its real
interest lies in its logical pattern, in the 'rapid and irresistible series of
deductions' it draws from the socialist polemics of France in its day,
couched in a 'simple and nervous' style.

Thiers's argument is more economic in its emphasis than Sudre's, less
political and ideological. The association of workers, he argues, or what
might later lead to collective bargaining, must prove inflationary, increasing
the price of goods and services as an effect of higher wages and salaries;
and inflation is always more likely to damage the interests of the poor
than of the rich. That prophecy does not now sound idle. Nor does Thiers's
view that a state-guaranteed right to work, which in 1848 some socialists
were demanding, could only lead in practice to the degradation of labour
by forcing skilled workers into unskilled jobs. The rights of a free people
are based on property, he concludes; and socialism, though less violent
than communism, must destroy liberty by destroying the rights of individ-
ual ownership. The difference, he argues, is only in style and tempo. 'The
Communists are pure utopians; the Socialists claim a more practical
character.' But their claim is an empty one. Socialism must depress the
living standards of the poor through inflation and destroy civil liberty too.

With the triumph of Gladstone in 1868 and, two years later, the fall of
Napoleon III, such sources as Thiers and Sudre were rapidly forgotten.
One reason was the failure of revolution itself. History had not marched to
the socialist drum. There were no class wars, only wars between nations.
The Paris Commune in 1871, like the Franco-Prussian war that had
precipitated it, found workers on both sides. Even Marx, in a speech in
Amsterdam in 1871, conceded that peaceful reform rather than bloody
revolution might, after all, be the way ahead, and long before his death in
1883 he had come to look harmless, while in Britain no socialist was elected
to the House of Commons until as late as 1892, with Keir Hardie, who sat
there alone.

As for literature, it is notable how little any writers of the last years of
the century, whether for or against socialism, refer to the great property
debate in the first exciting months of the Second French Republic of 1848.
Too much had happened since then. Erskine May, a clerk in the House of
Commons of Gladstonian sympathies, wrote an introduction to his
Democracy in Europe in 1877 where he called socialists and communists
'the most mischievous and dangerous fanatics of European democracy'.
But he did not suppose, as Thiers and Sudre had done nearly thirty years
before, that they were in any imminent prospect of taking power. John
Stuart Mill, another Gladstonian, had died four years earlier, in 1873, his
"Chapters on Socialism" (as they were called when they posthumously

appeared in the *Fortnightly Review* in 1879) uncompleted. The loss to radical literature is considerable, but Mill's case is clear enough in out-line, and the text has since been made fully accessible in his *Essays on Economics and Society*.

According to the preface of his stepdaughter, Helen Taylor, Mill conceived the work as early as 1869, provoked by the Second Reform Act of 1867 and the enfranchising in Britain of working-class voters. The United States moved towards manhood suffrage, too, in the late 1860s, after a civil war, a step first taken by France in 1848. Mill's task, then, was to educate the new masters of the electorate in much of the English-speaking world, conscious that socialist arguments might easily be made to look plausible to working people as they contemplated the manifest evil of 'great poverty, and that little connected with desert', along with the threat of a 'new feudality', as he strikingly calls it, of capitalists and entrepreneurs.

Nowhere does Mill mention Thiers or Sudre; his chief source in socialist literature is Louis Blanc's *Organisation du Travail* of 1839. During the Second French Republic Blanc had taken refuge in England, and Mill quotes his book extensively, refuting it point by point. Socialists tend to see only one side of competition, he argues – the side that depresses wages – and forget that capitalists, too, have to compete for commodities and skilled workers. In their hostility to private property, too, they forget that the concept is not fixed but variable: there are still states, after all, where slavery exists and where it is legal to own a human being, while in Britain 'we are only now abolishing property in army rank'. In other words, a competitive economy can and often does regulate and limit the powers of the rich. Communism, what is more, in abolishing the profit-motive, would encourage far bloodier instincts to flourish, so that equality of income would lead not to harmony but to violence. The labour theory of value, in any case, is an absurdity. The citizen who invests, Mill argues, is perform-ing a social service in forgoing for a period the use of his wealth, and it is fair as well as practical that he should be rewarded for doing so: 'As long as he derives an income from capital, he has not the option of withholding it from the use of others.' Labour, then, is not the only source of wealth.

Anti-property doctrines, in any case, Mill argues, are merely a muddle, since socialists commonly confuse the question whether the rich should invest their capital with the question whether they should possess it at all. But his real case against socialism is that it is reckless – rather as if he had anticipated the modern adage that the difference between socialists and scientists is that scientists try it on mice first:

> Those who would play this game on the strength of their own private opinion, unconfirmed as yet by any experimental verification, . . .

must have a serene confidence in their own wisdom, on the one
hand, and a recklessness of other people's sufferings on the other,
a recklessness, Mill adds, much like that of Robespierre and St Just in the
French Terror of 1793-4. Since Louis Blanc was openly an admirer of
Robespierre and the Jacobin tradition, the point is a telling one. Mill died,
however, leaving his critique of socialism unfinished and unpublished;
and Louis Blanc, who died soon after in 1882, a year before Marx, is
unlikely to have seen it. Events since then have supported Mill's view.
Both mice and men were experimented on, with the results he once feared.
He is a thinker still remembered and valued. But few, in the present century,
have had cause to mention Thiers, least of all his arguments in favour of
property, and nobody mentions Sudre. Perhaps the revolutionary Proudhon
was right, in 1848, to speak of platitudes. But he might have added that
the platitudes of one generation can be forgotten by the next and, in future
ages, regain their power to surprise.

7
Adolf Hitler

In April 1945, when Adolf Hitler died by his own hand in the rubble of Berlin, nobody was much interested in what he had once believed.

That was to be expected. War is no time for reflection, and what Hitler had done was so shattering, and so widely known in images of naked bodies piled high in mass graves, that little or no attention could readily be paid to National Socialism as an idea. It was hard to think of it as an idea at all. Hitler, who had once looked a crank or a clown, was exposed as the leader of a gang of thugs, and the world was content to know no more than that.

That mood, perhaps surprisingly, has lasted, and for half a century intellectual historians have commonly refused to take Hitler's mind seriously – J.P. Stern's *Hitler: the Führer and the People* (1975) being a notable exception – and have even dismissed inconvenient evidence in reported conversations as fabricated. There was a marked disinclination to dissect, and it started early. 'As to Hitler, I have no comment to make', the satirist Karl Kraus wrote as early as July 1933, fastidiously implying that the dictator was beneath his notice as a Viennese intellectual. Even the noisy *Historikerstreit* among German academics in the 1980s dealt more in bold assertions and surmises about his debt to Marxism than in textual evidence. The world, on the whole, did not want to know.

Half a century on, there is much to be said. Even thuggery can have its reasons, and the materials that have newly appeared, though they may not transform judgement, undoubtedly enrich and deepen it. Confidants of Hitler such as Albert Speer have published their reminiscences; his war-time table-talk is a book; early revelations like Hermann Rauschning's *Hitler Speaks* of 1939 have been validated by painstaking research, and the notes of dead Nazis like Otto Wagener have been edited, along with a full text of Goebbels's diary. If we prefer, for whatever reason, not to know the mind of Hitler and its sources, that is a matter of choice. But we can choose otherwise. The materials are there.

It is now clear beyond all reasonable doubt that Hitler and his associates believed they were socialists, and that others, including democratic socialists, thought so too. The title of National Socialism was not hypocritical. The evidence before 1945 was more private than public, which is perhaps significant in itself. In public Hitler was always anti-Marxist, and in an age in which the Soviet Union was the only socialist state on

earth, and with anti-Bolshevism a large part of his popular appeal, he may
have been understandably reluctant to speak openly of his sources. His
megalomania, in any case, would have prevented him from calling him-
self anyone's disciple. That has led to an odd and paradoxical alliance
between modern historians and the mind of a dead dictator. Like Karl
Kraus, many recent analysts have fastidiously refused to study the mind
of Hitler; and they accept, as unquestioningly as many Nazis did in the
1930s, the slogan 'Crusade against Marxism' as a summary of his views.
An age in which fascism has become a term of abuse is in any case un-
likely to analyse it profoundly.

His private conversations, however, though they do not overturn his
reputation as an anti-Communist, qualify it heavily. Hermann Rauschning,
for example, a Danzig Nazi who knew Hitler before and after his accession
to power in 1933, tells how in private Hitler acknowledged his profound
debt to the Marxian tradition. 'I have learnt a great deal from Marxism',
he once remarked, 'as I do not hesitate to admit'. He was proud of a
knowledge of Marxist texts acquired in his student days before the first
world war and later in a Bavarian prison in 1924, after the failure of the
Munich putsch. The trouble with Weimar Republic politicians, he told
Otto Wagener at much the same time, was that 'they had never even read
Marx', implying that no one who had failed to read so important an author
could even begin to understand the modern world; in consequence, he
went on, they imagined that the October revolution in 1917 had been 'a
private Russian affair', whereas in fact it had changed the whole course
of human history.[1] His differences with the communists, he explained,
were less ideological than tactical. German communists he had known
before he took power, he told Rauschning, thought politics meant talking
and writing. They were mere pamphleteers, whereas 'I have put into
practice what these peddlers and pen pushers have timidly begun', adding
revealingly that 'the whole of National Socialism' was based on Marx.
That is a devastating remark, and it is blunter than anything in his speeches
or in *Mein Kampf*; though even in the autobiography he observes that his
own doctrine was fundamentally distinguished from the Marxist by reason
that it recognised the significance of race – implying, perhaps, that it might
otherwise easily look like a derivative. Without race, he goes on, National
Socialism 'would really do nothing more than compete with Marxism on
its own ground'. Perhaps that remark is as near as he gets, in any public
statement, to acknowledging his Marxian debt. And at all such moments
an inner logic and consistency can be perceived through the untidy prose
of an untrained mind. He was not arguing to Rauschning or in *Mein Kampf*

1. Otto Wagener, *Hitler: Memoirs of a Confidant,* p. 167

that he was, or had ever been, a Marxist. He was arguing that National Socialism was based on Marx.

That claim, after all, is highly distinct. Many thinkers have based their beliefs on rejected systems of thought, and it is likely Hitler meant that he had done just that with Marx. Unlike his friend and ally Mussolini, he was not an ex-Marxist; from the first beginnings of his political career, as a returned soldier in the days of bitter defeat in 1918-19, he had been a dedicated anti-communist, and at a time when Germany came close to following Russia into a communist dictatorship. A pan-German nationalist, he had voluntarily joined the imperial German army, though still an Austrian, at the outbreak of war in August 1914; and since nationalism was always at the heart of his faith he could not call himself a Marxist. Marxism was internationalist. The proletariat, as the famous slogan goes, has no fatherland. Hitler had a fatherland, and it was everything to him.

And yet privately, and perhaps even publicly, he conceded that National Socialism was based on Marx. That, on reflection, makes consistent sense. The basis of a dogma is not the dogma, much as the foundation of a building is not the building, and in numerous ways National Socialism was based on Marxism. It was a theory of history, for one thing, and not, like liberalism or social democracy, a mere agenda of legislative proposals; and a theory of human history, not just of German, a heady vision that claimed to understand the whole past and future of mankind. A pure Nordic race, it proposed, had emerged untainted out of the subarctic regions in ancient times, hardened by climate into an ideal of heroic virtue, as if waiting to be celebrated in the operas of Richard Wagner. That is not a vision of history Marx would have recognised. But in the 1920s Marxism alone was the big picture, and it is easy to believe Hitler when he told Rauschning how, when he was young, 'and even in the first years of my Munich period after the war, I never shunned the company of Marxists'. They saw political action as struggle, and violent struggle, and if only for that reason their views must have excited him deeply. He even issued instructions to his party to admit communists unquestioningly into its ranks. 'The petit bourgeois Social Democrat and the trade union boss will never make a National Socialist, but the Communist always will', he told Rauschning. Politics for them, as for Hitler, meant an élite fired by a single-minded theory of the past and future of mankind and claiming an exclusive right to power because it, and it alone, understood the way the world must go.

Hitler's discovery, in those postwar years, was that socialism could be national as well as international. There could be a national socialism. That is how he reportedly talked to his fellow Nazi Otto Wagener in the early 1930s. The socialism of the future would lie in 'the community of the Volk', not in internationalism, he claimed, and his task was to 'convert

the German Volk to socialism without simply killing off the old individ-
ualists', meaning the entrepreneurial and managerial classes surviving from
the age of liberalism. They should be used, not destroyed. The state could
control, after all, without owning; guided by a single party, the economy
could be planned and directed without dispossessing the propertied classes.
That realisation was crucial. To dispossess, after all, as the Russian civil
war had recently shown, could only mean Germans fighting Germans,
and Hitler believed there was a quicker and more efficient route. There
could be socialism without civil war.

Now that the age of individualism had ended, he told Wagener, the
task was 'to find and travel the road from individualism to socialism
without revolution'. Marx and Lenin had perceived the right goal, in other
words, but chosen the wrong route – a long and needlessly painful route –
and, in destroying the bourgeois and the kulak, Lenin had turned Russia
into a grey mass of undifferentiated humanity, a vast anonymous horde of
the dispossessed; they had 'averaged downwards'; whereas the National
Socialist state would raise living standards higher than capitalism had
ever known. That, in the event, was not an altogether empty boast. Within
two years of taking office a large programme of public investment,
combined with a lucky upturn in the trade cycle, created 2.3 million new
jobs in Germany through public expenditure on roads, railways and other
public utilities along with munitions and house-building, stimulating the
economy beyond the most hopeful predictions. While Russia languished
in famine, Germany prospered and rearmed; and Bismarck's tradition
of state welfare since the 1880s helped to make such programmes look
patriotic and German. In July 1943, for example, the Nazi journal
Signal greeted the Beveridge Plan for a British health service with
open disdain, contrasting the belated British response to poverty with
what it proudly called 'the sixty-year-old historical development of
socialism in Germany since 1883', when Bismarck introduced his
workers' contributory health scheme. The Nazi article is called
"Socialism in Action", and it implies that social welfare is a practice
long since pioneered in Germany, and that Germans act while others
prate.

It is plain that Hitler and his associates meant their claim to socialism
to be taken seriously and that they took it seriously themselves. As early
as April 1934, for example, Richard Walther Darré, Hitler's minister of
food and an eminent apologist of the new régime, announced that Jewish
political theory, whether conservative, liberal or socialist, had always been
dedicated to mere self-interest (*Ichsucht*), whereas the socialism of Adolf
Hitler was corporate. The argument insists that totalitarianism is itself a
kind of socialism:

> The socialism of Adolf Hitler's National Socialism is starkly
> opposed to such Jewish notions. It is the structured order of a whole
> people according to its own laws of life, and its concept of state is
> its method of guaranteeing and strengthening that order.[1]

Marxist influences were wide and deep. If the age of individualism was
dead, so was the notion of objective knowledge – a bourgeois illusion,
Hitler told Rauschning, useful to professors in its day but to be swept
aside once education became an instrument of a one-party state. Democracy
was effete, the transient creation of a nineteenth-century optimism that
Marx and Darwin had forever demolished. They had provided a new scien-
tific basis for the government of mankind, whereby whole species must be
swept aside if they do not meet the demands of history. The sanctity of
human life was the mere sentimentality of a dying age; mankind, like the
factories, mines and fields, can henceforth be scientifically planned. Hitler's
mind was as futuristic as Lenin's and as atheistic and republican, some-
times in astounding ways. In 1976, for example, in *Spandau*, Albert Speer
tells how in January 1943 Hitler had expressed a lively admiration for
communists who had fought in the Spanish civil war, deriding 'that
reactionary crew around Franco' who wanted to restore an ancient social
order and a Catholic monarchy. All the idealism in Spain, he told Speer,
had been with the Reds, and one day he would begin the Spanish civil war
all over again and 'with us on the opposite side', fighting shoulder to
shoulder with the communists against the forces of reaction.

For half a century, none the less, Hitler has been portrayed, if not as a
conservative – the word is many shades too pale – at least as an extreme
instance of the political Right.

It is doubtful if he or his friends would have recognised the description.
His own thoughts gave no prominence to Left and Right, and he is unlikely
to have seen much point in any linear theory of politics. Since he had
solved for all time the enigma of history, as he imagined, National Social-
ism was unique. The elements might be at once diverse and familiar, but
the mix was his.

The claim that Hitler was right-wing, in any case, is riddled with
inconsistencies. It is said that he was too lazy to read books through, least
of all a difficult book like Marx's *Capital*, though the same might be said
of many socialists, Marxian and non-Marxian, both before and since. It is
said he took money from capitalists, but so did Lenin; and that he was
hostile to new ideas in the arts, though Stalin was too. It is not usually
denied that Lenin and Stalin were socialists, and it is hard to suppose that

---

1. R.W. Darré, *Um Blut und Boden: Reden und Aufsätze,* pp. 291-2

those who parade such arguments can seriously believe in them. Socialists have often been too lazy to read Marx, have often been artistic conservatives and been subsidised by the rich. There are no grounds here for denying that Hitler was a socialist.

The notion that National Socialism was significantly indebted to big business, in any case, has recently been refuted. In *German Big Business and the Rise of Hitler*, Henry Ashby Turner, in a well documented study, has shown that Hitler received relatively little support from big business before he came to power in January 1933, in spite of many blandishments, and that his party grew during the late 1920s and after largely as a self-financing body, without any significant aid from large-scale enterprise. Its chief centre was Bavaria, in any case, which was mainly agricultural, and big business in the Weimar Republic had reasons to be hostile, or at least suspicious, after the failed Munich putsch of 1923. Nazism was tainted with illegality, after all, and its economic programme, although calculatedly ambiguous, smacked of anti-capitalism in some of its elements.

Like Marxism before it, Hitler's doctrine saw itself as a science rather than a sect. In its own unquestioning view, National Socialism stood above and beyond any influences that he might acknowledge in conversation. It was above and beyond Left and Right, rich and poor, Protestant and Catholic. It offered itself as the expression of an entire nation and an entire people. Its propaganda, as in the Horst Wessel song, even-handedly vilified Reds and reactionaries, and its public claim from first to last was to have ended forever the divisions of bickering churches and parties that had debilitated a great people and made its borders the easy prey of greedy neighbours. Germany would unite under one dogma and one leader. That dogma was socialist in its insistence on a command economy, national in that it excluded no one who was judged to be truly German. Bolshevism, its only serious competitor as a radical ideology, it supposed to be as backward and incompetent as everything Slav must be, offering encouragement only in its ruthlessness. Stalin was a genius, as Hitler casually remarked in his table-talk in July 1942, at the height of a war against his old ally, because he had seen that politics meant action and a contempt for the rules. Marxism had definitively shown the world where history was going; and Hitler, as he once told Rauschning, was Marx's executor: he would carry his prophecy through to the end. But he was always certain there were quicker and better ways to arrive at the promised land than the communist way.

Hitler's mind, it has often been noticed, was in many ways backward-looking: not medievalising, on the whole, like Victorian socialists such as Ruskin and William Morris, but fascinated by a far remoter past of heroic virtue. It is now widely forgotten that much the same could be said of

Marx and Engels. Engels's late writings on kinship extolled an age before written documents when, as he believed, mankind was not yet cursed with private property. Marx's *Ethnological Notebooks*, recently edited from manuscripts in Amsterdam, show the same fascination with prehistory, when mankind had not yet been corrupted by private greed. Socialism from the start had looked backwards as well as forwards. In the*Communist Manifesto* Marx and Engels had represented the bourgeoisie as crudely and dangerously radical; by building factories and railroads and debasing human relations to a sordid cash-nexus, it had 'stripped of its halo every occupation hitherto honoured and looked up to with reverent awe' and 'torn away from the family its sentimental veil'. That sounds like a lament for family ties, a call to respect the authority of tribal elders; and three years before, in *The Condition of the Working Classes in England*, Engels had bitterly attacked capitalism for forcing women into factories where, as he darkly hinted, they became the sexual prey of managers and foremen. Traditional family virtues mattered greatly to the early socialists; they had no patience with liberal values such as free love. Hitler's notorious view that women should be guardians of the home and dedicated child-minders may sound conservative now, but it may not have been conservative in its origins. It was all there in the socialist traditions of an earlier century which, as he often told his friends, were an essential study to anyone who sought to understand the modern age.

But it was the issue of race, above all, that for half a century has prevented National Socialism from being seen as socialist. The assumption that socialism was never racist can now be seen as a misunderstanding.

The proletariat may have no fatherland, as Lenin said. But there were still, in Marx's view, races that would have to be exterminated. That is a view he published in January-February 1849 in an article by Engels called "The Hungarian Struggle" in Marx's journal the*Neue Rheinische Zeitung*, and the point was recalled by socialists down to the rise of Hitler. It is now becoming possible to believe that Auschwitz was socialist-inspired. The Marxist theory of history required and demanded genocide for reasons implicit in its claim that feudalism, which in advanced nations was already giving place to capitalism, must in its turn be superseded by socialism. Entire races would be left behind after a workers' revolution, feudal remnants in a socialist age; and since they could not advance two steps at a time, they would have to be killed. They were racial trash, as Engels called them, and fit only for the dung-heap of history.

That brutal view, which a generation later was to be fortified by the new pseudo-science of eugenics, was by the last years of the century a familiar part of the socialist tradition, though it is understandable that since the liberation of Auschwitz in January 1945 socialists have been eager to forget it. In 1902 H.G. Wells concluded his *Anticipations* with a programme of socialist genocide, and Franz Mehring, a German Marxist who in 1902 had edited the Engels article of 1849, echoed the point with qualified approval in his life of Marx of 1918. In the United States, meanwhile, Jack London (1876-1916), the Californian socialist whose writings would one day fascinate the young Orwell and Lenin on his death-bed, had independently arrived at a similar conclusion, combining revolutionary socialism with white-supremacist views in what a recent reviewer has called 'a strange mixture'. It would not have seemed strange, however, at the turn of the century. Jack London believed in Darwin as well as in Marx, and Darwinian theories of evolution, he held, demanded the triumph of the fittest proletariat on earth, which of course was white. 'The lesser breeds cannot endure', he wrote defiantly in a letter of 17 April 1899. 'I cannot but hail as unavoidable the Black and the Brown going down before the White.' This is socialist imperialism at its most full-blooded; and as the *S.S. Oregon* returned to San Francisco from the war with Spain, when the US annexed the Philippines and Cuba, London hailed it rapturously on behalf of the Hearst press in the *San Francisco Examiner* of 14 June 1901:

> Up, up she swept, grandly on the breast of the flood tide, this huge
> gun platform, this floating fort, this colossus,

praising her great guns as 'teeth which have tasted' and recording 'the hot blood' that rushed at the sight back through centuries of mere civilisation to a darker and more potent age, 'things primordial and naked'. Tomorrow the lion may lie down with the lamb. 'But today it were well that we look to our *Oregons* and see that they be many and efficient.' That was written within months of H.G. Wells's appeal for socialist genocide in *Anticipations*, and doubtless in ignorance of it.

Ethnic cleansing was orthodox socialism for a century and more. 'By the same right with which France has taken Flanders', Engels wrote in the *Neue Rheinische Zeitung* of 10 September 1848, as well as Alsace-Lorraine, and will soon take Belgium, 'by that same right Germany takes Schleswig: with the right of civilisation against barbarism, of progress against stability'. That, as he believed, was the supreme right, 'worth more than all treaties, for it is the right of historical development'. Havelock Ellis saw it as part of the essential socialist quest for white racial purity. Capitalism believes in mere quantity, both in terms of goods and in terms of people; socialism, by contrast, in quality: 'the question of breed, the production of fine individuals, the elevation of the ideal of quality in human production over that of mere quantity' – a noble ideal in itself, and also 'the only method by which socialism can be enabled to continue on its present path'. That is from Ellis's *Task of Social Hygiene* of 1913, which unites Marx's early vision of inevitable class conflict with eugenic theory and the coming triumph of the white races.

Sidney and Beatrice Webb echoed the point in the same year in the *New Statesman*. If the higher race, as they call the whites, were to lose their world predominance through a falling birth rate, there would be a cataclysm in which they would be replaced by a 'new social order developed by one or other of the coloured races, the negro, the Kaffir or the Chinese'. That prospect made the Webbs ultra-imperialists:

It would be idle to pretend that anything like effective self-government, even as regards strictly local affairs, can be introduced for many generations to come – in some cases, conceivably never (2 August 1913).

So the socialist intelligentsia of the western world entered the first world war publicly committed to racial purity and white domination, and no less committed to violence. On 16th December 1939, after the partition of Poland by Hitler and Stalin, Hewlett Johnson, Dean of Canterbury, defended what Stalin had done, though not on the grounds Stalin had offered. He should, the Dean wrote in the *New Statesman*, have simply said: 'We are trustees for the world's first Socialist State.' It was a word that justified, by then, any action whatever. Since there is no morality but class morality, G.D.H. Cole wrote in the same journal after the war, 'it was therefore justifiable and necessary for the proletariat to use any method, and to take any action, that would help it towards victory over its class-enemies'.

Socialism offered a blank cheque to violence, and its licence to kill included genocide. In 1933, in a preface to *On the Rocks*, for example, Bernard Shaw publicly welcomed the exterminatory principle which, to his profound satisfaction, the Soviet Union had already adopted. Socialists could now take pride in a state that had at last found the courage to act, though some still felt that such action should be kept a secret. In 1932 Beatrice Webb remarked at a tea-party what 'very bad stage management' it had been to allow a party of British visitors in the Ukraine to see cattle-trucks full of starving 'enemies of the state' at a local station. The account is predictive, nearly ten years before the Nazis began their own mass deportations at the height of the second world war. 'Ridiculous to let you see them', said Beatrice Webb, already an eminent admirer of the Soviet system. 'The English are always so sentimental', adding with assurance: 'You cannot make an omelette without breaking eggs.' The story was recorded years later by her niece, Konradin Hobhouse, in a letter to the *Manchester Guardian* in February 1958, and it makes plain that some socialists knew of the Soviet exterminations as early as 1932 and accepted, even welcomed them as an essential part of a socialist programme. Such ideas were not limited to dictatorships. A few years later, in 1935, a Social Democratic government in Sweden began an eugenic programme for compulsorily sterilising gypsies, the backward and the unfit, and continued it till after the second world war.

The claim that Hitler cannot really have been a socialist because he advocated and practised genocide suggests a monumental failure, then, in the historical memory. Only socialists in that age advocated or practised genocide, at least in Europe, and from the first years of his political career he was proudly aware of the fact. Addressing his own party, the NSDAP, in Munich in August 1920, he pledged his faith in socialist racialism:

> If we are socialists, then we must definitely be anti-semites – and
> the opposite, in that case, is Materialism and Mammonism, which
> we seek to oppose.

There was loud applause, and the young Hitler went on promptly to accept the challenge of answering how one could be both a socialist and an anti-semite: 'How, as a socialist, can you not be an anti-semite?'[1]

The point was widely understood, and it is notable that no German socialist in the 1930s or earlier ever sought to deny Hitler's right to call himself a socialist on grounds of racial policy. In an age when the socialist tradition of genocide was familiar, that would have sounded merely absurd. The tradition, what is more, was unique. In the European century that began in the 1840s, from Engels's article of 1849 down to the death of Hitler, everyone who advocated genocide called himself a socialist, and no exception has been found.

The first reactions to National Socialism outside Germany are now largely forgotten.

They were highly confused, for the rise of fascism had caught the European Left by surprise. There was nothing in Marxist scripture to predict it, and it must have seemed entirely natural to feel baffled. Where had it all come from? Harold Nicolson, a democratic socialist and after 1935 a Member of the House of Commons, conscientiously studied a pile of pamphlets in his hotel room in Rome in January 1932 and decided judiciously that fascism (Italian-style) was a kind of militarised social-ism; though it destroyed liberty, he concluded in his diary, 'it is certainly a socialist experiment in that it destroys individuality'. The Moscow view that fascism was the last phase of capitalism, though already proposed, was not yet widely heard.

Shortly afterwards, in 1933, another British socialist, Julian Huxley – Aldous Huxley's brother and, after 1946, the first director-general of

---

1. Adolf Hitler, *Sämtliche Aufzeichnungen 1905-24,* pp. 200-1

UNESCO – issued a signed statement that unwittingly echoed Harold Nicolson's point. An eminent biologist who admired the Soviet system, he saw fascism as an unwelcome distraction; 'a short cut towards the unified Socialised State which should be our goal' and hence dangerously oversimplified: 'its methods are so crude that it is likely to land us in war and social disaster, while delaying real progress.' No attempt here to deny that fascism was part of the wider family of socialist ideas, though plenty of embarrassment about its details. It was the black sheep of the socialist family. Next year Julian Huxley returned to the point in *If I were a Dictator*, writing now with Hitler firmly in the saddle in Germany. 'A crude system', he called it, and 'a despairing attempt to find a short cut to the promised land. . . . .' None of these comments are imperceptive; it is clear that National Socialism was not yet seen as conservative or right-wing, and Huxley makes no attempt at that early stage to deny that Hitler's name for his movement was a broadly accurate one. He saw in Hitler a sort of violent caricature of what socialists believed, and his deeper concern was that the dictator might give socialism a bad name. That seems to have been the provisional view of Richard Crossman, too, who in a 1934 BBC talk remarked that many students in Nazi Germany believed they were 'digging the foundations of a new German socialism'.[1]

That view was not to last. By the outbreak of civil war in Spain, in 1936, sides had been taken, and by then most western intellectuals were certain that Stalin was Left and Hitler was Right. That sudden shift of view has not been explained, and perhaps cannot be explained, except on grounds of argumentative convenience. A single binary opposition like cops-and-robbers or cowboys-and-Indians is always satisfying. Even the German-Soviet alliance of August 1939, shattering as it was, did not shake the new terminology. The Molotov-Ribbentrop pact was seen by hardly anybody as an attempt to restore the unity of socialism, and that claim was not made for it even in Moscow or Berlin. A wit at the British Foreign Office is said to have remarked that all the Isms were now Wasms, and the general view was that nothing more than a cynical marriage of convenience had taken place.

By the outbreak of world war in 1939 the idea that Hitler was any sort of socialist was almost wholly dead. One may salute here an odd but eminent exception. Writing as a committed socialist just after the fall of France in 1940, in *The Lion and the Unicorn*, Orwell saw the disaster as 'a physical debunking of capitalism'; it showed once and for all that 'a planned economy is stronger than a planless one', though he was in no doubt that Hitler's victory was a tragedy for France and for mankind. The

---

1. Anthony Howard, *Crossman: the Pursuit of Power*, p. 42

planned economy had long stood at the head of socialist demands; and National Socialism, Orwell argued, had taken from socialism 'just such features as will make it efficient for war purposes'. Hitler had already come close to socialising Germany: 'Internally, Germany has a good deal in common with a socialist state.' These words were written by a British democratic socialist just before Hitler's attack on the Soviet Union, and Orwell believed that Hitler would go down in history as 'the man who made the City of London laugh on the wrong side of its face' by forcing financiers to see that planning works and that an economic free-for-all does not.

At its height, Hitler's appeal transcended party division. Shortly before falling out with him in the summer of 1933, Otto Wagener heard him utter sentiments that would eventually be published after his death in 1971 as a biography by an unrepentant Nazi. Wagener's *Hitler: Memoirs of a Confidant*, composed in a British prisoner-of-war camp, did not appear until 1978 in the original German, to be issued in English, without much acclaim, as recently as 1985. Hitler's remembered talk offers a vision of a future that draws together many of the strands that once made utopian socialism irresistibly appealing to an age bred out of economic depression and cataclysmic wars; it mingles, as Victorian socialism had done before it, an intense economic radicalism with a romantic enthusiasm for a vanished age before capitalism had degraded heroism into sordid greed and threatened the traditional institutions of the family and the tribe.

Socialism, Hitler told Wagener shortly after he had seized power, was not a recent invention of the human spirit, and when he read the New Testament he was often reminded of socialism in the words of Jesus. The trouble was that the long ages of Christianity had failed to act on the Master's teachings. Mary and Mary Magdalen, Hitler went on in a surprising flight of imagination, had found an empty tomb, and it would be the task of National Socialism to give body, at long last, to the sayings of a great teacher: 'We are the first to exhume these teachings.' The Jew, Hitler told Wagener, was not a socialist, and the Jesus they crucified was the true creator of socialist redemption. As for communists, he opposed them because 'basically they are not socialistic'; they created mere herds, Soviet-style, without individual life, and his own ideal was 'the socialism of nations' rather than the international socialism of Marx and Lenin. The one and only problem of the age, he told Wagener, was to liberate labour and replace the rule of capital over labour with the rule of labour over capital.

These are highly socialist sentiments, and if Wagener reports his master faithfully they leave no doubt about the conclusion: that Hitler was an unorthodox Marxist who knew his sources and knew how unorthodoxly he handled them. He was a dissident socialist. His programme was at once nostalgic and radical. It proposed to accomplish something that Christians had failed to act on and that communists before him had attempted and bungled. 'What Marxism, Leninism and Stalinism failed to accomplish', he told Wagener, 'we shall be in a position to achieve'.

That was the National Socialist vision of history. It was an exciting vision, at once traditional and new. Like all socialist views it was ultimately moral, and its economic and racial policies were seen as founded on universal moral laws. By the time such conversations saw the light of print, regrettably, the world had put such matters far behind it, and it was less than ever ready to listen to the sayings of a crank or a clown.

That is a pity. The crank, after all, had once offered a vision of the future that had made a Victorian doctrine of history look exciting to millions. Now that socialism is a discarded idea, such excitement is no doubt hard to recapture. To relive it again, in imagination, one might look at an entry in Goebbels's diaries. The day was 16th June 1941, five days before Hitler attacked the Soviet Union, and Goebbels in the privacy of his diary exulted in a victory over Bolshevism that he believed would quickly follow. There would be no restoration of the Tsars, he remarked to himself, after Russia had been conquered, for he was as sturdy a republican as his master. But Jewish Bolshevism would be uprooted in Russia and 'real socialism' planted in its place. *'Der echte Sozialismus. . . .'* Goebbels was a liar, to be sure, but no one can explain why he would lie to his diaries. And to the end of his days he believed that socialism was what National Socialism was about.

8
Marx and the Holocaust

Awaiting execution in 1947 in a Polish prison, Rudolf Hoess composed his memoirs, and in *Commandant of Auschwitz* he recalled how even at the height of the Nazi-Soviet war of 1941-5 his Nazi colleagues had respected the Soviet example of an exterminatory programme based on forced labour. The Nazis had known that programme in 1939-41 as Soviet allies, if not earlier, and after their attack on the Soviet Union in June 1941 they grew more impressed than ever by the sheer scale of its camp system, in evidence gathered mainly from escapees: so much so that Nazi camp commandants were sent detailed reports, Hoess recalled, admiring above all the Soviet readiness to destroy whole categories of people through forced labour:

> If, for example, in building a canal, the inmates of a camp were used up, thousands of fresh kulaks or other unreliable elements were called in who, in their turn, would be used up.

The reference is tantalisingly thin, but the Soviet example was evidently felt to inspire, even to justify, as a precedent, what Hoess at Auschwitz did.

Since 1945, however, little has been heard of the Nazi debt to the Soviet camps. This is partly out of postwar respect for an ally, and partly the result of a surprisingly effective act of censorship that has only recently come to light. With the defeat of Hitler, Stalin became gravely concerned about revelations of Nazi-Soviet collaboration during the joint occupation of Poland in 1939-41, and it is now known that he put Vyshinsky in charge of a secret commission to guide the conduct of war-crimes trials at Nuremberg and to prevent such information from being made public.[1] The Soviet state knew it had a lot to hide.

That revelation makes it easier to realise that the totalitarian idea knowingly grew from a common source, attracted (often enough) the same thinkers, and exchanged ideas and even techniques, both as allies and as opponents in war. Anti-semitism is one aspect of a far wider issue here – the issue of genocide, or killing by category. Its movement from Left to Right in France, with the Dreyfus affair of the 1890s, has been well charted, the French Left abandoning anti-semitism around the turn of the century, mainly because the Right chose that moment to take it up.[2] The French

---

1. Arkady Vaksberg, *The Prosecutor and the Prey,* pp. 298-9
2. Zeev Sternhell, *La Droite Révolutionnaire 1886-1914*

Socialist Party publicly and conscientiously dissociated itself from the Dreyfus affair; on 19th January 1896 its parliamentary party, including Jean Jaurès, issued a manifesto published the next day in *La Petite République*, calling it a power-struggle within the ruling class and warning the workers against taking sides, on the dogmatic grounds that many Dreyfusards were Jewish capitalists. It refused to recognise injustice or to condemn it.

The incident prefigures exchanges between fascism and communism in the coming century, where similar positions might easily be confessed in private and disowned in public. The common sources here go as far back as the 1840s, and by the 1940s the extermination of whole races had been an element in socialist thought for a century. Genocide was an idea unique to socialism. Engels had called for it in January-February 1949 in an article on the Hungarian war that Marx published in his journal the *Neue Rheinische Zeitung*. The article, often applauded and translated, was commended by Stalin in *The Foundations of Leninism* of 1924. Several years earlier the German Marxist Franz Mehring in his *Life of Marx* had praised its general tenor, as a friend of Engels, though in a passage that remains faintly obscure he dissented from Engels's specific programme, which had concerned Serbs and other Slavs, as well as Basques, Bretons and Scottish Highlanders:

> Engels was wrong when he denied any historical future to the smaller
> Slav nations, but the fundamental idea which governed his attitude
> was undoubtedly correct (VI.3),

he remarks laconically, having summarised Engels's article at some length. Mehring, who was a friend and comrade of Rosa Luxemburg and Franz Liebknecht, died shortly after, in January 1919, a week or so after their brutal murder in Berlin, and at a moment when a number of small Slavic nations were about to be created; as a German, like Marx and Engels, he may have felt that the notion of a fragmented self-determination in former Hohenzollern or Habsburg lands was silly or worse. It is unlikely we shall ever know for certain what he meant when he praised Engels's fundamental idea about the extermination of small nations, while querying its details, but his close acquaintance with Engels's 1849 article is not in doubt, since he had edited it in a collection called *Aus dem literarischen Nachlass von Marx, Engels und Lassalle* – the collection where, in all likelihood, Stalin and Hitler found the doctrine of Marxist genocide in its original form.

What was that form? It was, from first to last, a power-worshipping idea, for Marx and Engels were only interested in winners. The bourgeoisie was about to lose to the proletariat, as they believed, in a worldwide workers' revolution; but an obsession with class war and a fervent belief in economic determinacy did not exclude race. 'We regard economic conditions as that which ultimately determines historical development', Engels wrote to W. Borgius in January 1894, 'but race is itself an economic factor'. And so, given the white-supremacist assumptions of the founders of Marxism, it plainly was. A few years previously, in his "Notes to Anti-Dühring", Engels had observed that the inheritance of acquired characteristics extended the argument from the individual to the species:

> If, for instance, among us mathematical axioms seem self-evident to every eight-year-old child, and in no need of proof from experience, that is solely the result of 'accumulated inheritance'. It would be difficult to teach them by proof to a bushman or to an Australian negro.

The whites, in the Marxist view, are the bearers of progress. Among the whites, big peoples like the Germans and the Russians are superior – simply because they are big – to small nations and ethnic remnants like Bretons, Basques and Serbs. 'The Poles as a nation are done for', Engels wrote to Marx on 23 May 1851; they have achieved nothing except a 'brave, quarrelsome stupidity'. Russia, on the other hand, is 'really progressive in relation to the East', a civilising influence on the Black Sea, the Caspian Sea and in central Asia. That is a highly imperial vision of history. Engels's conclusion was 'to take away as much as possible from western Poland', presumably by planting it with German settlers, and 'to occupy her fortresses, especially Posen, with Germans, under the pretext of defence'; as for the rest, 'to let them make a mess of things, to drive them into the fire, to eat up their country. . . .' Hitler is unlikely to have read the correspondence of Marx and Engels; but if he had read that letter, he might have cheered loudly. He might also have cheered a passage from "Revolution and Counter-Revolution in Germany", in the *Neue Rheinische Zeitung* in March-April 1852 – an article signed by Marx but probably written by Engels – condemning to extinction the French and Spanish creoles recently conquered in the Americas by the Anglo-Saxon race, and 'those dying nationalities the Bohemians, Carinthians, Dalmatians etc.', who need to accept the blunt verdict of a thousand years of history: that 'such a retrogression is impossible'. They should accept 'the physical and intellectual power of the German nation to subdue, absorb and assimilate its ancient eastern neighbours'. That, after all, is how civilisation has spread. The British conquest of India, and the United States conquest of California, are praised in the same journal, and in similar terms.

The brutality of that programme was its proudest boast, and Marx and Engels would have been puzzled by any attempt to deny that they were dedicated to conquest and extermination. That audacity of utterance was perhaps their chief legacy to Stalin and Hitler. It has nothing to do with